AN
INTRODUCTION
TO
MEDICAL AUTOMATION

AN INTRODUCTION TO
MEDICAL AUTOMATION

L. C. PAYNE, BSc, PhD
*Formerly Director, Medical Automation Unit,
University College Hospital, London*

P. T. S. BROWN
*Formerly Manager, Medical Automation Unit,
University College Hospital, London*

Second Edition

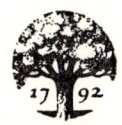

J. B. Lippincott Company
Philadelphia   Toronto

First Published 1966 in Great Britain by Pitman Medical
Second Edition 1975

ISBN 0-397-58153-X

Library of Congress Catalog No. 74-15388

Published in North America
by J. B. Lippincott Company
Philadelphia Toronto

© L. C. Payne 1966, 1974 and P. T. S. Brown 1974

Printed in Great Britain by
The Whitefriars Press Ltd, London and Tonbridge

Contents

Preface		vii
1	Computers and Automation: Basic Principles	1
2	The Concept of Automation	15
3	A Brief History of Computer Development	24
4	The Features of a Data Processing System	34
5	Communications and Networks	51
6	Medical Records Procedures	55
7	Computer-assisted Diagnosis	74
8	Computer-assisted Measurement, Analysis and Communication	99
	APPENDIX 1. How the Computer Works	115
	APPENDIX 2. Natural Binary	140
	Glossary	143
	Index	157

Plates

Between pages 40–41
Plate 1
- A Transferring data sheets to punched form
- B A Piece of punched paper tape
- C Paper tape keyboard punch

Plate 2
- A A Punched card keyboard punch
- B A paper tape reader
- C A card reader

Plate 3
- A Magnetic ink character reader
- B Optical character reader
- C A paper tape punch

Plate 4
- A Card punch
- B Line printer

Between pages 48–49
Plate 5
- A A Graph plotter
- B A Visual display unit

Plate 6
- A Magnetic tape unit
- B Magnetic disc unit

Plate 7
- A Magnetic tape driving off-line printer
- B View of Technicon Auto-Analyzer

Plate 8
- A Pen recorder and Auto-Analyzer
- B Ferrite cores

Preface

THE INCREASINGLY pervasive influence of the computer in modern society and, in particular, in the health care services, is much more apparent today than when the first edition of this book appeared in 1966. Then, the idea of computer-assisted patient management, ward management, clinic management, and so on, was regarded, when considered at all, as a repugnant interference in what were essentially human activities quite unsuited to any form of mechanisation. Today, however, there is a growing awareness of new horizons of opportunity opened up by the advent of the computer in terms of both increased logistic efficiency and enhanced medical effectiveness, particularly in the clinical management of the patient. There is also, a growing awareness that the ability of the computer to assist, replace and generally augment trained cerebral activity is as important as its ability to perform calculations. Since the health services are highly dependent on brain power—some 70 per cent of the considerable expenditure on these services being disbursed in wages and salaries—then the main effect of the advent of the computer is the prospect of achieving greater effectiveness and productivity by means of capital-intensive procedures in many sectors which currently are highly labour-intensive.

Inevitably such a trend must have a radical effect on the organisation and objectives of traditional practices, and it is vital, if the integrity of medicine in relation to its purposes and practices is to be maintained, that the staffs of all health care organisations (doctors, nurses, administrators, and others) understand the nature of the forces at work, and participate actively in bringing about the necessary changes. Only harm can come from blind opposition, from blind acceptance, or from abdicating responsibility to others 'who know about these things'.

This book is a modest attempt to arouse the interest of the general medical reader in a subject that will inevitably affect all who are involved in the care of patients and who undertake research. At the same time, it carries a message, which is, that computers are too important to be left to the expert, be he computer scientist or medical computer enthusiast. This truism is so flagrantly and constantly neglected that we make no apology for its repetition throughout the text.

L. G. PAYNE
P. T. S. BROWN

Acknowledgements

The authors wish to thank the following for the loan of photographs and permission to reproduce them in this book:
Burroughs Machines Ltd
Computer Technology Ltd
Computer Weekly
International Computers Ltd
Sanaca Computing Services
Scientific Furnishings Ltd

I
Computers and Automation: Basic Principles

THE FIRST POINT to be emphasised about a computer is that it is a *machine*, just as a refrigerator or a motor-car is a machine. To say, as is often said, that it is 'stupid', or 'intelligent', or 'decides what to do', is a misconception. Yet one has to acknowledge that while such things are said about computers, they are not said about other machines, and in order to explain in what way a computer is unique some description must be given to the functioning of other machines.

Machines with which most of us are familiar have one essential common feature: they enable muscle-power to be deployed more effectively. They can for example *assist* muscle: typewriter plus muscle is more effective than muscle alone; motor-car plus muscle is much more effective than muscle alone; but in both cases muscle-power is required to direct the use of the machine. They can *replace* muscle, as they do in the case of the automatic dishwasher or thermostat. Most important of all, they can do things that no amount of combined muscle-power could ever achieve: like jet engines transferring hundreds of tons at hundreds of knots, or manufacturing plant producing millions of screws, buttons, pills, or newspapers a day. Hardly any of this could have been conceived when James Watt produced his steam-engine two hundred years ago. Comparing his simple reciprocating piston with the subtlety and dexterity of their own fingers, those who doubted at the time that such a simple if powerful device would displace manual craftsmanship may possibly be forgiven. A feat of intellectual comprehension was needed to see that systems of gears and linkages could be designed to 'programme' the right amount of power into the right place at the right angle; to see that the machines which would displace manual craftsmanship would not, and could not, simulate the physiology of muscle-power; and to foresee that the material wealth of nations would be determined principally by the machine-power *per capita*.

The key feature of this so-called first industrial revolution in fact is *the separation of designing and making* (inextricably interwoven in the manual craftsmen), so that those who can design and create, do, and those who cannot, make (with machine assistance). A well-designed machine for making a button, a telephone component, or a tumbler embodies the knowledge and experience of the designer in such a way that unskilled or semi-skilled operators, with the aid of power-driven jigs and tools, can produce not only what earlier craftsmen tried to make, but other things they could not make at all: think only of tin cans, bottles, motor-cars and television sets produced at low prices and in large quantities. The idea of machines assisting, replacing and extending muscle-power is a fact of common experience; it does not offend our vanity to use them; in fact, few of us could, or would want to live at all without machine-power, and not to use it would be regarded as either primitive or unintelligent.

A MACHINE THAT ASSISTS, REPLACES AND AUGMENTS CEREBRAL FUNCTION

What has been achieved and accepted in relation to machine-power and muscle can now be achieved, if less readily accepted, in relation to computer power and cerebral function. Thousands of tasks which at present require trained or semi-trained brain-power, such as many clerical, administrative and mathematical procedures, can already be performed more effectively by computers; and throughout this book we shall highlight numerous examples where this is already so in the health and medical services. But this is only a beginning. Many who contemplate the simplicity of the computer mechanism, described in detail in Appendix 1, may be forgiven for doubting that such a simple if powerful device could possibly replace *mental* craftsmanship, the know-how and experience of managers and professionally qualified people, doctors, nurses, or administrators. A feat of intellectual comprehension is needed to see that programmed data-procedures, described below, can assist, replace and, most powerfully of all, refine and extend the application of brain power in the management of patients, departments and hospitals;

but to see, also, that the computer that will do this will not, and cannot, emulate the physiology of cerebral function. Modern societies based on machine-power are dependent on trained man-power at every level—clerks, operators, supervisors, technicians, controllers, managers, lawyers, doctors and architects—for their efficient functioning. As this trained man-power steadily and inevitably becomes computer-assisted, the wealth of such societies will come to be as directly correlated with computer-power *per capita*, as it already is with machine-power *per capita*. The key feature of this second industrial revolution, as it has come to be called, is the *separation of knowledge and experience from the performance of an increasing number of intelligent activities* (inextricably interwoven in the mental craftsmen), so that those who have the knowledge and experience to formulate intelligent procedures will do so, and those who have neither ability nor training will implement them quickly and accurately (with computer-assistance).

The idea of machines assisting, replacing, and extending brain function is not a fact of common experience, and at this stage it usually offends human vanity to be 'replaced by a computer', but we are rapidly moving in a direction where not to use computer-power, to rely exclusively on naked brain-function alone, will soon be regarded as either primitive or unintelligent. A radical reorganisation of professional work and practices is presaged by these developments in medicine, education, administration and management comparable to the reorganisation of manual skills that was required to effect the first industrial revolution. The analogy we have drawn between manual skills and machine-power, and brain-skills and computer-power, is neither false nor exaggerated, and the task to which we must now address ourselves is to establish the credibility of this perhaps surprising point of view.

In general terms a computer is a machine with four attributes—

(*a*) information (or data—the terms are used synonymously) can be put into it ('input');
(*b*) such information can be stored in it;
(*c*) the stored information can be automatically operated on by it;
(*d*) stored information can be printed out or transmitted ('output') from it.

The first, second and fourth of these properties are quite unexceptional: a handbag, a desk-drawer, or any filing cabinet have similar properties. It is the third property, the ability automatically to process data stored in the machine, that uniquely differentiates it from all previous storage devices; in fact it may be regarded as an active file rather than a passive file.

We therefore need to concentrate on the computer's unique ability to process data. This is all that any computer can do, but considerable elaboration is required to bring out the significance of these words. In order to carry out a data procedure, a computer must evidently be supplied with two things; the data and the procedure, in some suitable form (discussed at length later). Once this is done, on pressing the start button of the computer the procedure is caused to operate on the data, giving rise to a resultant action which will depend entirely on the data and the procedure.

TABLE I

Data	Procedure	Action of Computer
1. Numerical	Arithmetic	Calculation
2. Dictionaries	Syntax	Translation
3. Musical Notes	Harmony	Composition
4. Chess positions	Rules	Play
5. Traffic densities	Rules	Traffic Control
6. Electrocardiograph	Rules	Diagnostic Indication
etc.	etc.	etc.

A few out of many possibilities are listed in Table 1. If, for example, the data supplied to a computer is numerical in character, and the procedure is arithmetical in character, then the computer's action in applying the arithmetical procedure to the numerical data will be to calculate. In the simplest of situations the data might relate to hours of works and rates of pay, and the procedure might describe how to calculate gross pay and net pay after tax deductions; the computer's action in this case would correspond exactly to that of a payroll clerk, a job which, before the introduction of computers, could be performed only by a trained clerk. Thus, as is well known, computers can compute, and hence they have a considerable role to play in carrying out a host of arithmetical procedures arising in subjects as diverse as astronomy and molecular biology, the design of roads and aircraft, meteorological forecasting, and so on.

One example in this category that arises in medicine, and to which computers have been successfully applied, is that of radiation treatment planning. In applying a lethal dose of radiation to malignant tissue, a great deal of careful calculation is required to prepare a suitable pattern of radiation which minimises the dose given to the unaffected tissue and delivers a lethal dose to malignant growth. This subject is discussed in greater detail later. The important point to note here is that, before computers, this was an exclusively mental activity which could be performed only by skilled personnel with adequate training and experience. Now that a suitable computer procedure exists, however, someone without training, using the computer procedure, can produce a competent treatment plan. Even more to the point, someone without training, and even without the ability to be trained, may produce a competent treatment plan.

This is a point of the utmost significance in the concept of being computer-assisted. The normal cycle of human endeavour is that a fresh mind takes over a job knowing little about it, but with training and experience acquires a certain level of competence dependent on intrinsic ability. Subsequently, some circumstance removes the person from the job and an accumulated amount of knowledge and experience is commonly lost, or at least must be relearnt by the next incumbent. But if, while a person is at his peak level of competence, we induce him to set down his knowledge in such a way that it is embodied in a computer procedure, then this knowledge will be preserved. The neophyte, using nothing more than a button-pressing procedure, will be practising with this degree of competence *from the start*, and only if his intrinsic ability is such as to enable him to become more competent than his predecessor will he be in a position to do better than the computer procedure. And in this case, of course, he will be in a position to modify and improve the computer procedure that he initially took over. It must be admitted, however, that not every process is suitable to be performed by computer.

A number of important general consequences ensue from this.

Firstly, we see that computer procedures enable us to consolidate knowledge and experience which would otherwise, when located in cerebral units alone, be lost. Secondly, we are enabling each new person to add his own improvements to what existed before. This is a long-standing practice elsewhere. For example a jet engine, an internal combustion engine, a television set, or a typewriter is never designed by one person but by hundreds of designers. Each generation of designers adds their little bit, so that increasing performance and sophistication are possible. Only rarely do exceptional mortals appear to reject improvement by modification and to propose new principles instead, as when Einstein altered our basic thinking about space-time, or Whittle brought in a new concept of the aero-engine. Because most computer procedures operating today are first-generation models, the additional advantages of improvement by modification are still to be reaped as time goes by. A third consequence is that the existence of a computer procedure provides an explicit standard of operating practice that can be inspected and discussed by others; this is a notable advance over personal and private performance. A fourth consequence, as observed earlier, is that the existence of a computer procedure enables certain persons (operators of limited abilities who only operate the drills) to do to a known standard what, without computers, they could never do at all. Fifthly, creative, thinking people, who originate useful computer procedures, can be liberated from carrying them out without fear that standards of practice will fall; they will have more time to think and to refine. Straight economic comparisons that do not take cognisance of these factors are missing the most important ingredients in the equation. All the manual craftsmen that ever existed could not possibly produce the volume of goods that are produced by unskilled and semi-skilled operators today, with machine assistance. The creators, as we have said, design the jig and tools, the operators and technicians produce the goods. Is it too far-fetched to call a computer procedure a 'cerebral jig' which, once designed, enables modestly skilled operators to produce first-class results of a known standard? Is it too elementary to suggest that thinking should be separated from doing, or too fanciful to contemplate that by the year 2000, all the mental craftsmen that ever lived could not supply the skilled assessment and decision procedures which will by then be made in abundance by semi-skilled and unskilled computer-assisted operators? As we have remarked, the role of computers in performing data-procedures is by no means confined to calculation, which happens to be one particular kind of data-procedure. If, to take an entirely different example (*see* Table 1), the data supplied to a computer is (*a*) two vocabularies, say those contained in the English and Russian dictionaries, and (*b*) a Russian text, and if the computer procedure embodies the rules of syntax in these two languages, then the computer's action in operating the procedure on the data might be to translate the text. The standard of translation will, of course, depend entirely on *how well the rules have been formulated in the procedure,* and this, in turn, will depend primarily on the linguistic skills that have been employed. The computer can no more be blamed for a bad translation than it can be applauded for a good one. The machine is neither stupid nor intelligent; it has no more idea of the semantics of the procedure it is performing than a washing machine has of the colours of the garments it is handling: both are carrying out a prescribed sequence of operations. How such a sequence is carried out by a computer is described in detail in Appendix 1. Of course, there is a limit to how far even the best of linguists can formulate rules of translation, and this is what sets the absolute limit to which computer translation is possible. What is certain, however, is that a good linguist will probably formulate good rules, and a bad linguist will probably formulate bad rules. However, too often, the task is left entirely to a computer specialist who has no specialist linguistic knowledge, producing indifferent results.

The moral of this is that the design of effective computer procedures cannot be left to computer scientists alone—throughout this book we have repeatedly emphasised this point—good linguistic procedures require good linguistic knowledge; good cardiological, psychiatric, obstetric procedures, and so on, require good cardiological, psychiatric and obstetric knowledge. But how often is the task handed over by the specialist to the 'computer chap'; certainly his skills are needed for reasons that we shall explain in due course, but he cannot by himself produce good computer procedures for subjects in which he is not trained. The computer is neither intelligent nor stupid; it simply carries out the instructions given to it, and if there are omissions, even obvious omissions, they will be dealt with literally, dutifully, and mercilessly. Most so-called computer errors are, in fact, human errors in designing computer procedures or programs. It is worth pointing out, however, that once such errors are discovered and corrected, the program is corrected once and for all, whereas in human practice the rare event, due to unfamiliarity, will often be overlooked or dealt with incorrectly, although some events can readily be corrected by human common sense, which the machine totally lacks.

Musical notes, to take another example, are finite in number and may be coded suitably into a computer as data. Rules of harmony, especially of the modern duodecatonic type, exist and may be incorporated in a computer procedure, so that when the start-button is pressed, the computer, by operating the procedure on the data, can produce a musical composition, which in more advanced applications can be made to control ('play') a variety of instruments to produce tunes. Not the most obvious use perhaps of a 'data-processing' machine, i.e. a computer, but one, nevertheless, that has exercised the energies of a number of computer-minded musicians in recent years.

DATA-PROCEDURES THAT EXHIBIT INTELLIGENCE AND LEARNING CHARACTERISTICS

Another example, illustrating other basic principles with powerful potential uses in a wide variety of situations, may be taken from chess. It is a straightforward matter to supply a computer with data indicating the positions of each chess piece: BK (5.4) for example would amply indicate that black knight was at five across and four down. In addition, we can supply the computer with a directory indicating for each possible configuration of the chess pieces the moves that first-class players would consider. Such a directory would be extensive, and would take many years to compile (and for this reason most chess-playing computer procedures adopt a rather different approach which avoids the need for such a directory); in paper form it would certainly occupy thousands of cubic feet, but stored in a computer (in a way described later) it would be very compact indeed. The data then consists of (*a*) the positions of the chess pieces updated after each move, and (*b*) an extensive directory listing first-class moves for each and every configuration. A possible computer procedure might be as follows—

(*a*) scan the directory to ascertain what moves are possible;
(*b*) select one of these moves at random.*

Since a modern computer could carry out this procedure in seconds, and since its action would consist of 'playing' first-class moves at random, it would clearly be an effective 'player'. The effectiveness, however, *does not depend on intelligence*, but on the ability of the computer to store millions of first-class moves (which even the ablest chess-playing individual cannot) and access them incredibly quickly (which the ablest chess-playing individual cannot). The reader will appreciate that this procedure could, in principle, be implemented manually, that is without a computer, but it would not be very practical for a player to say to his opposite number, 'excuse me for a year while I go and look up the directory'. There is a story that, before computers, the meteorological office had an excellent way of calculating a four-hourly weather forecast, but it used to take some twelve hours to work it out! It is doubtful, therefore, that it was used very often. Once twelve hours is reduced to twelve seconds then a useless method becomes useful, and the incentive exists to refine the method further. Modern molecular biology, requiring hundreds of man-years of calculation to elucidate protein structures, could not have achieved the remarkable progress it has without the use of computers. Medicine, too, might benefit from following a similar approach to the chess-playing procedure described above, since medical diagnosis and treatment rest essentially on the ability of clinicians to identify a patient as belonging to one or other of more than 30,000 treatable categories continually being refined and extended. The effectiveness of medicine as currently practised is fundamentally limited by the knowledge of these numerous categories that a single doctor can memorise. In effect, the clinician is saying to the patient: 'either you belong to one of the few hundred treatable categories I know of, or you're fit, or you might try to fix up consultations in one or more of the thirty-odd other medical specialties to see if your particular illness can be identified'. The situation is not helped by the fact that clinicians are confident because they are not aware of the extent of their own ignorance.

*Random procedures, such as that employed in the United Kingdom by ERNIE to select winning premium bonds, are easy to arrange.

The art, and it is an art, of diagnosis, treatment and prognosis is that of making important, sometimes critical decisions, on all too little information. Without computers this limitation has to be accepted, but a growing number of clinicians are beginning to recognise the possibility of systematically compiling a medical directory of differentiating syndromes and treatments, which might be telephoned to 'to see what moves are possible'.

The chess-playing example allows further refinement, using a technique that has many potential applications elsewhere. Any chess player knows that certain moves work better against some players than others, and quickly learns to take advantage of the fact. Some of this learning ability may be incorporated into the computer procedure; all one needs to do is to insert into the computer additional data pertaining to the relative success of particular moves against particular players. This shows that in a situation, say, where one of three moves is possible, each move is weighted by the accumulated frequency of its success on previous occasions. In effect, the directory stores ('memorises') not only what moves are possible, but also the frequency of success of each move against particular players, which, of course, is merely quantitative data. The computer procedure now becomes—

(a) scan the directory to ascertain what moves are possible;
(b) select one of these moves at random *taking account of weighting factors*.

If such a computer procedure were designed, it would clearly be possible for its designer reasonably and honestly to assert that, 'although I designed the procedure, I do not know which particular move the computer will choose; I only know that it will be a first-class move, taking account of what happened in previous games against this particular player'. This example should amply illustrate—

(a) why anthropomorphisms abound in describing a computer's actions;
(b) why a computer's action can appear intelligent or stupid (depending on the design of the procedure it is carrying out) although it is neither;
(c) why a computer is only limited in what actions it can perform by what procedure can be devised for it to carry out (which

is as open-ended as saying a piano can play anything that can be composed);
(d) why an untrained person, computer-assisted, can perform as well as a trained person.

One final example will illustrate other basic principles and terminology which are specially relevant to both patient monitoring and laboratory automation. Consider the familiar problem of traffic congestion. Most readers will have experienced this problem at first hand, and will also on occasion have said to themselves, 'if I'd known about this a mile back I would have gone round the other way'. In the vicinity of most areas of congestion there is a way round if only one had the information, but relying on the physiological senses alone one has insufficient information to make the choice; thus information, or usually the lack of it, restricts decisions. Or, think of the phenomenon of the 'police assisted congestion'. A police officer controlling an intersection, limited in what he can see by the density of the traffic, is equally limited in what he can do to resolve it. If he is operating in a rural area at an isolated intersection, then, because outside the immediate area of the intersection there is ample road space, he can clear the situation reasonably well, but if he is operating in an urban area he may well be clearing traffic into the same areas as one of his colleagues at the next intersection. It is not his fault: like the clinician in a diagnostic situation he can only do as well as the information at his disposal allows him to, and this is cerebrally limited.

But now suppose, without using a computer at this stage, that all the police officers are removed from the intersections to a control room, and let us suppose that they are all looking at a map which is animated by a traffic pattern compiled from automatic sensing devices, which count the traffic, in each street of the given area. At least they will benefit, in switching the traffic signals, by having more information in front of them. The trouble is, however, that it may take them time, perhaps several minutes to decide what to do, because the rate at which a number of people can assess a situation and make decisions takes time. Hence, the next step is to insert the map, or rather the information contained on it, into a computer and have it (at electronic speeds) evaluate the situation and 'decide what to do', according to criteria and rules applied to it in the form of a computer procedure. This is the essential basis of computer-assisted traffic control; it is also the basis of computer-assisted control in oil-refining, steel-making, and many other industries, as well as in operating theatres, recovery rooms, and intensive care units; instruments automatically and continuously supply information to a computer, which applies assessment and decision rules built into its procedures.

In such situations, of course, there is not sufficient time for the data to be physically transported to the computer; it must be *directly connected* to the computer by electrical means, and commonly this is achieved by using the telephone system to transmit the data. This is what is meant by saying that the computer is 'on-line': the data must be fed to the computer at the rate at which it is changing. Equally important, the intrinsic speed of the computer must be fast enough for it to assess the data and make decisions at the rate at which the situation is changing: in the above case of traffic control this probably means re-assessing the data about every minute. A computer operating in this mode is said to be working in 'real-time', i.e. at the speed at which the 'real' situation is developing; hence, the jargon 'on-line real-time data-processing'. This is in contrast to 'off-line' data-processing, such as pay-roll calculations, engineering calculations, and so on, where it is usually acceptable for the data to be supplied to the computer at times which are much less critical in terms of urgency. The computer is then said to be operating in 'batch' mode.

From even the small number of examples that have been cited, it should be apparent that computers are not simply machines confined to carrying out routine arithmetical and clerical chores. In effect, they are capable of modelling many decision processes, which, in their purely cerebral mode, whether it be translation, musical composition, chess-playing, traffic control, diagnosis, and so on, are characterised by being at least partly subjective and intuitive, and certainly qualitative. Such are the attributes of mental and manual craftsmanship. Just as the latter were systematised into machine procedures harnessing artificial sources of energy, so we are beginning to see that the former may be systematised into computer procedures or programs. Progress is rapid, but in relation to what will be achieved within the next generation the process has hardly begun. The idea ingrained in most of us, namely that only human beings can exhibit intelligence and judgement (because prior to the computer all actions pertaining to assessment, judgement and decision *necessarily* and *exclusively* involved the human mind) must change. It no longer makes sense to refuse to call 'intelligent' today that which a computer can now perform, when yesterday we called it intelligent when only we ourselves could perform it. A computer's *actions* can be as intelligent as the procedure it is carrying out.

The outlook that must be acquired by all wishing to use computers, is that of endeavouring to systematise at least some of our thought processes in terms of data-procedures. Those now being educated will doubtless find this more natural than those who have already achieved status as mental craftsmen. It is not obvious, nor indeed natural, for most people to see chess-playing, or diagnosis, or radiation treatment planning, or meteorology, or dietetics, as data-procedures. The knack has to be acquired. For example, though the reader may never have thought of it, the intelligent action of a thermostat in maintaining a uniform temperature is effected by carrying out a data-procedure. The thermostat in fact is an 'on-line real-time data-processing' machine. It collects one piece of data continuously, namely current temperature, and it simply compares this temperature with a pre-set temperature, using a bi-metal strip (which expands/contracts differentially with temperature) as its small self-contained computer; its 'output' switches the heater on or off. In a manner of speaking we could say that 'it knows when to switch the heat on and off'; 'it is deciding what to do'—but we don't regard it as an 'intelligent' competitor with ourselves. We would all acknowledge that the cheapest thermostat can, twenty-four hours a day, day in, day out, maintain a far more uniform temperature than can any human being, i.e. that it exceeds the performance of its designer, yet none of us believe that we are going to be taken over by thermostats. But many people believe they are going to be taken over by computers because computers exceed the performance of their designers. Of course they do; all machines exceed the performance of their designers, which is why they are invented, but no new principle is embodied in the computer that is not present in the thermostat. It is a matter of degree; instead of subjecting one piece of data to one single comparison, a computer has the ability to deal with many pieces of data, and subject them to much more complicated procedures. Computers, however, are *not* brains, or anything like brains. It so happens that one useful function of the human brain (but by no means the only one) is the ability to perform data-procedures. A machine has now been invented that can perform data-procedures better, faster and more cheaply than human brains. No more than that, but equally no less than that. Intelligent people will enlist its services in mental processes, just as they enlist machine-power in physical processes.

A man who has never owned a motor-car can readily argue that he does not need one: 'I never go more than a few miles'. And, indeed, if he only used the motor-car to travel the one and two-mile journeys that he travelled before acquiring it, it would not make much sense economically or otherwise to buy one. Those readers with a motor-car, however, will know that the new dimension of mobility afforded by it opens up new opportunities, makes accessible relationships and ways of living that would otherwise be impossible. At this time, understandably, a great deal of computer-power is being used simply to carry out the one or two-mile cerebral processes that we are used to doing, rather than exploiting the new dimension of opportunity that it makes possible. As this potential is realised the mental craftsman, manager, doctor, teacher, lawyer, as we know him today, will be displaced, as the manual craftsman was displaced by machine-power. In broad terms, just as machine-power successively and steadily reduced the numbers required to produce enough food for the community, and steadily increased the numbers engaged in manufacturing enterprise with machines, so with computers and automation the proportion engaged on managing, controlling and supervising, on assessing, judging and deciding the operations of everyday life will be successively and steadily reduced: machines —self-monitoring, self-diagnosing, self-adjusting and self-maintaining—will do it better. An increasing proportion of the population will be involved in service activities, servicing the old and the young and the infirm, servicing leisure and education, and servicing patients.

2
The Concept of Automation

WE HAVE NOW ARRIVED at the point where we can explain what is meant by *automation*. In common currency few words have a wider or looser connotation: it has been used at one time or another to describe every piece of mechanisation that man has had the ingenuity to contrive, and since mechanisation of one sort or another has been with us for centuries many intelligent people wonder what all the fuss is about. They seriously question whether it means anything more than the progressive elimination of chores and routine tasks by highly repetitive machine systems which replace individual craftsmanship and personal service by a limited range of standard products and services. On this understanding, of course, the very notion of *medical* automation is repugnant.

This, however, is to misinterpret the essential nature of automation. *Automation is not mechanisation*, which is essentially the application of machine-power to deploy muscle-power more effectively. *Nor is* automation to be equated simply with computers. Computers, as we have seen, are machines for carrying out data-procedures, and when, for example, they perform routine clerical tasks or complex calculations, they are merely mechanising these functions. One of the results of an insufficient grasp of the basic concept of automation is that computer-power may be too strongly directed to the simple mechanisation of existing paper procedures, thus perpetuating in electronic equipment the limitations of 'handraulic' methods of management and administration. Computers are essential for the achievement of automation, but in any large-scale system of automation, and medical automation will be no exception, typically the computer element will constitute a small part of the whole. What then is automation if it is not to be equated simply with mechanisation or computers? A brief, precise definition is certainly possible and will be given in due course, but if this definition is to be understood clearly, some explanation may be helpful.

The first industrial revolution was initiated by the advent of steam power. The capital cost of the generating equipment, as well as its size, precipitated the birth of the factory; and the very limited means by which steam power could be applied, namely through some form of rotary action, necessitated the breaking down of manual procedures (such as weaving for example) into sequences of elementary and highly repetitive operations. These were often of the most boring character from the point of view of the human operators, as all that each of them needed to do to his particular piece of equipment was to stop it, start it, load it, unload it, grease it, and perhaps adjust it occasionally; the process as a whole was no concern of individual machine operators. Unhappily, this type of work organisation is still to-day most commonly employed in factories, although significant changes have been introduced in some major industries. Clerical work, too, as most readers know, follows a similar pattern in large organisations: each clerical unit carries out a particular drill, and passes its results on to the next clerical unit for further drills to be performed, and so on.

During the two centuries, from 1760 to 1960, the main addition to this method derived from the advent of electric power and the internal combustion engine. Each of these sources of energy became available in a wide range of power units, so that whether one wants to shave, dry one's hair, or drive a ship or an aeroplane an appropriate unit is available. This, as we have already seen, has its counterpart in computer-power, which is already available in a wide range of units from match-box size (in missiles) to very large installations, so that it is pointless to talk of the speed and size of a computer without reference to a particular machine and its purpose. Also, it should be noted that the main effect of the availability and the harnessing of other sources of energy was not just to reproduce a more economic standard of life of the type that existed at the time of its introduction in 1760, but rather to redeploy the displaced workers in creating an extraordinary variety of industries which could not have been previously imagined. We may confidently expect that computer-power, too, will have similar extensive repercussions.

During the 1920s, at the great Ford motor plant in Detroit, machinery was introduced to detect automatically when one operation was complete, and to transfer automatically the work to the next operation, thus largely displacing individual human operators. The entire process was then said to be 'automated'. Such a regime is excellently suited to performing the particular set of operations involved, being both highly efficient and robot-like, but it is *not* automation. Its very excellence for the particular sequence of operations involved makes it useless for any other; it has no capacity for adaptation. In fact, it is what we may call *fixed-strategy mechanisation*, because it is only capable of performing a particular, or fixed, operating strategy. To overcome this inflexibility, an obvious extension is to design for each stage machines that have more than one mode of operation as well as possibly a continuous range such as would be provided by an adjustable screw. By choosing a particular mode of operation for each machine, any one of a variety of operating strategies could be selected. This obviously gives the system some flexibility, since it is not committed for ever to only one operating strategy, but once a particular selection has been made and an operating strategy chosen, the regime is once again robot-like in character until some manual interference selects a different operating strategy. This we shall call multiple-strategy mechanisation, emphasising that it is still mechanisation; it is not automation.

To proceed to the next step we must reflect carefully on the considerations and events that influence the changeover from one operating strategy to another. Whatever situation one is trying to manage, be it an aircraft in flight, a patient undergoing treatment, or the production of some marketable commodity, the factors determining the situation seldom remain constant for long. In the manufacture of a product the market requirements may change, there may be some variation in the quality of the raw materials, there may be some wear in a machine part, and so on. In flight there may be changes in wind direction, changes in altitude dictated by traffic requirements, changes in temperature and pressure affecting engine performance, changes in load as fuel is consumed, and so on. In treating patients, there may be new symptoms or signs or new test results which may necessitate changes in treatment; changes in diagnosis are also not infrequent. All this is the very stuff of management, which essentially involves initiating action in response to awareness of what is happening—but if one is not aware of what is happening, no action, or the wrong action, will be initiated. Action is circumscribed by information. We have therefore to consider in detail how changes in any particular situation are brought to notice, and how they lead to changes in management or operating strategy (i.e. action). The following cycle is usually involved—

1. observation   ⎫
2. measurement   ⎬ data collection
3. recording   ⎭
4. transmission   data communication
5. assessment   ⎫ data analysis/comparison/
6. decision   ⎬ prediction
7. re-transmission   data communication
8. action

The first three steps, observation, measurement and recording, are obviously of prime importance since they set the limits to our awareness of the situation we are trying to manage. Herein lies one of the commonest limitations of what may be called our 'eyeball-cerebral' faculties, the limited accuracy and frequency with which we can observe and record changes in one or a number of variables characterising any particular situation. This fact contributes to the fragmentation and division of labour among human beings (even in medicine a history is taken here, a test there, an X-ray somewhere else, treatment, surgery, and so on). Tasks are tailored to the capacity of an individual to assimilate and deal with what is going on, so that no particular individual is aware of the whole developing situation. Each individual can only do the best he can with such information as he has at the time that decisions are required. If this is less than the best that could be done, it is usually not because of any lack of interest but because he cannot be aware of, let alone assimilate, all that is relevant to the management of the whole. Therefore, in many situations, the 'operators' (the people actually carrying out the operations) filter some information back to a supervisory body, but it is only *some* of the information. Once again it has to be tailored to what the supervisory body can assimilate about the whole process. In addition, communication delays and inaccuracies lead to all manner of decisions being taken on out-of-date and incomplete information to a degree dependent on the speed and complexity of the process involved. Man's ability to sense accurately and continuously what is going on in any management situation is obviously severely circumscribed. By comparison, instrument systems (especially those connected to computers) work much more efficiently as, being aware of many more changes in a situation than an unaided brain, the possible responses (management actions) are improved. They can be programmed to read dynamically.

This, however, is only the first part of the 'decision data-cycle'. The following stages of data assessment, evaluation and decision highlight other limitations of the eyeball-cerebral faculties, namely the ability to assimilate, analyse, compare, and correlate all the relevant data to arrive at the 'best' or optimal decision, *in the time available for decision-making.* Seldom is this done quantitatively, seldom is it done with any precision, and for those who argue that it never can be, perhaps the chess-playing procedure described earlier may convince them. 'Experience counts' of course, but this is simply a way of saying that decisions are hardly ever made from current information alone. Whether a situation is satisfactory or not may often only be determined in relation to previous situations, and this is limited by our unawareness of many relevant past situations and the limited experience of any one individual. One of the outstanding features of computers is their capacity to store (and check the accuracy of) a prodigious amount of information or data collected from a variety of sources that in aggregate can far exceed human memory capacity, and then to retrieve from this store of information selectively, according to set criteria in a particular situation. This does not necessarily mean handing over decision-making to the machine; it is using computer-power to enable many more factors to be taken into account than a human brain can assimilate and retain. How many important decisions are taken based on too little information and in too short a time? Errors arising from taking decisions using too much information, a tendency to be avoided with computers, are hardly likely to exceed those arising from using too little.

Enough has probably been said for it to be appreciated that the process of decision-making consciously or unconsciously involving all the steps in the data-cycle has serious deficiencies in terms of old and incomplete information. These deficiencies are inevitable in unaided human decision-making, but may be lessened to some extent by technological assistance. It is clear that the entire decision-making process in changing from one operating strategy to another may take hours, days, or weeks, depending on what consultations, information, and even what committees have to be marshalled together. If, however, all stages of the information-loop are fully instrumented, and especially if this is done electrically, the business of changing from one operating strategy to another may be speeded up by a factor of a thousand or more. Moreover, such a system will respond automatically to a greater variety of changes in the operating situation than the unaided human senses could possibly be aware of. A regime of this sort will be called *adaptive mechanisation*. It is *not* robot-like, quite the contrary. This is *automation*.

The crux of the automation process, therefore, is not mechanisation but information; without information flow there can be no adaptive potential. Automation of any complexity has had to await the advent of the computer, because previously there were no means of instrumenting information, or of carrying out by machine the relevant data-procedures. The computer, therefore, is a vital part of any automation system. A concise definition of automation can now be given:

AUTOMATION MEANS INSTRUMENTING INFORMATION
FOR DECISION OR ADJUSTMENT PURPOSES

In effect, automation is *built-in management*. It not only includes physical actions by machines, whether for productive or clerical purposes (mechanisation), but essentially involves collecting information on these actions in order to determine if they are achieving their objectives, and to adjust the system accordingly.

Before concluding this chapter, it might be helpful to classify automation systems according to their complexity. Perhaps the simplest example is that of the thermostat; a simple bi-metal strip that is set to open when a pre-determined temperature has been reached, and close when the temperature reduces again. Temperature is the only variable. Only two management actions are possible: switching the heater on or off. The objective is clear—to maintain a uniform temperature. In this case the information-loop reduces to a single-channel; compare with a pre-set temperature; signal on or off. All the ingredients are there in this simplest of information-loops, which we shall call a *single-channel closed-loop information system*. It is fully instrumented, and the situation is fully automated. It can do what a human-being cannot; namely, respond to changes to which the human senses are insensitive, and it can do this continously without pause for rest. A modern digital computer was not needed to automate this situation, because the data-procedure (a simple comparison) could be achieved by using a bi-metal strip. It upsets no one that 'it exceeds the performance of the designer'; it upsets no one to say of it 'that it is deciding what to do'. It embodies all the basic principles of automation; it happens that the system objective, the information loop, and the decision criterion are all very simple. The most advanced computer-based automation systems differ only in degree in the relative complexity of their objectives, their decision criteria, and the number of variables contained in the situation being managed.

In more complex situations, such as air conditioning plant, oil refining, baking, and steel-making for example, it is necessary to maintain many variables at pre-set levels. This may be accomplished by using independent single-channel closed-loop information systems: that is, in addition to a thermostat, there might be what we will call a 'flowstat', a 'humidity-stat', or a 'level-stat'. The total information loop in this case consists of a number of independent single-channel loops; there is no interaction between them. In still more complex situations, such as homeostasis, or in maintaining an aero-engine at optimum efficiency, it may be less important to keep constant each variable than to maintain *relationships* between variables. In this case the information-loop is more complex: several pieces of information need to be collected, the correlation between them determined, and adjustment to several variables may be necessary to maintain the correlation.

Finally, there will be those situations where 'experience counts', where the data-profile of several variables characterising a situation (for example, a differentiating syndrome) will need to be compared with memorised (stored) profiles to ascertain which is the most relevant (diagnosis) and, hence, retrieve the appropriate adjustments (treatments). The information procedures in such cases, and they apply to most higher-level decisions outside medicine as well as inside it, are relatively more complex, and considerably greater ingenuity may be required to work out suitable information algorithms.* The chess-playing example given earlier indicates that solutions are possible in unfamiliar situations.

So far, we have implied that the entire information-loop (data measurements, assessments, decisions and so on) can be fully instrumented, but in practice this is not generally true. Where it is true, as in certain chemical, steel and oil-refining processes (or in the case of the thermostat), the human operator has no useful part to play. But where it is not true, as in most aspects of clinical and surgical activity, in flying, and in many types of management decision, even the fullest information that can be instrumented has very often to be weighed against intangible or human factors that cannot at present be measured, and that perhaps never will be measurable. In these cases, computer-evaluation will not lead directly to decisions, but must be presented for human assessment. A good example of where this is already achieved is in the cockpit: no pilot can continuously and efficiently monitor all the information presented to him on the numerous dials that confront him, but a computer can pre-digest a major part of it continuously and alert the pilot's attention to any trend that may require his attention. Automation, although *partial,* is still extending the cerebral faculties without assuming complete control. A host of situations in medicine may be similarly aided by partial automation, where computers regularly, if not continuously, digest certain information from medical records, medical instruments, prescription forms, and surveys to reveal significant happenings requiring early action, and significant correlations which otherwise would not be revealed. In addition, there are other means of instrumenting medical data so that diagnosis, therapy and prognosis are made on the basis of adequate information.

It is essential that the proper 'interface' is established between the man-machine system so that the integrity of decision is preserved, although the evidence on which it is based is substantially improved. The following chapters indicate some of the developments in medical automation made possible by these new tools and concepts. Even if not all the possibilities are realised at once, and this is unlikely, there can be little doubt that everyone

---

*An algorithm is a set of rules and criteria completely specifying the method.

working in medicine will be greatly affected as his or her functions are re-assessed and new procedures introduced.

It will be clear that the scope and nature of medical automation may be assessed from a systematic examination of the many different uses that are made of *information* in medicine, especially relating to *management*, whether clinical or administrative. The application of automation to finance, accounting or administration will not be dealt with since the practices and systems required are already well covered elsewhere. Suffice it to say that hospital and health administration, while it remains technologically unaided, is doing 'handraulically' and expensively what could be done more cheaply. More importantly, it is not managing in any dynamic sense; it is confined to doing this year more or less what was done last year. Hospital administration is not based on up-to-date information of what has actually just happened but on outdated and incomplete information of what happened days or weeks before. Significant changes can and do happen without the administration being aware of them, and while this may not be without its advantages, it does not lead to effective administration.

3
A Brief History of Computer Development

It is a remarkable fact that throughout the whole of history prior to 1946, the year in which the first ever electronic digital computer, the ENIAC, was launched, the only machines capable of processing data were desk calculators (originated by Pascal and Leibnitz in the seventeenth century, but not in commercial production until the early nineteenth century); punched card apparatus (originated in the late nineteenth century by Hollerith in the U.S.A.) whose operations were limited to sorting, counting, and tabulating; and special calculators (originated about 1930) capable of solving some types of mathematical equations. Most tasks involving data therefore, whether for administration, management, control, assessment or decision, *necessarily* and *exclusively* involved the human mind; it alone was capable of intelligent action. While two centuries of machine-power, applied on an increasing scale and with increasing sophistication, have radically altered the tempo and complexity of government, commerce and industry, the decision-making processes to direct and manage this complexity were, prior to 1946, almost entirely dependent on the speed and capacity of the unaided cerebral cortex.

It was into this situation that the ENIAC was launched, and it was, as we have seen, a machine uniquely different from any previous machine, in that it was not concerned with assisting, replacing or extending human muscle, but with assisting, replacing and extending cerebral function, that is, with deploying brain-power more effectively. It could perform what previously only human brain-power could perform; namely, the carrying out of a great variety of data-procedures by means of a stored program. This alone would have made the ENIAC a historic innovation, but coupled with it was its capacity to carry out these data-procedures *a thousand times faster* than a human being—a capacity which not only augured a thousand-fold increase in output by the computer-assisted cerebral cortex, but also the capacity to accomplish many tasks that would otherwise be impossible, like simulating new hospitals and airports before they were built, controlling whole regions of road, sea and air traffic more safely and more rationally, making well-organised 'libraries' of knowledge and experience more readily available, and signalling control data from satellites. Also, there was the prospect of global communication for distributing not only news, pictures and entertainment, but also, eventually, educational and professional advice and consultation, and streamlining bureaucracies (sluggish brain empires) so that administration was more informed, flexible and more tolerant of detail.

ENIAC was an engineering *tour de force*: it weighed some thirty tons and it comprised some 18,000 valves which, between them, generated as much heat as 150 one-bar electric fires. Statisticians, working on their knowledge of the life-cycle of one valve, calculated that 18,000 of them could not possibly work at the same time, but, as even statisticians should know, rare things not only do happen but they *must* happen with precisely the small probability assigned to them. And so ENIAC had its moments, and was intensively nursed by teams of skilled engineers for these apocalyptic outbursts, each of which produced the equivalent of many man months of trained cerebral activity, and each of which by its rarity and novelty provided banner headlines for newspapers throughout the world. ENIAC *was* gigantic, and it *was* performing brain-like actions, and inevitably therefore, was referred to as a 'giant brain', an understandable misnomer perhaps, but one which contributed not a little to a considerable amount of misunderstanding. Today, little more than twenty-five years on, computers more powerful than ENIAC are commercially available for less than £10,000, which occupy less space than a cubic foot, and which require only as much power as an electric lamp. The first step in this direction was made in 1947, when John von Neumann, working at Princeton, U.S.A., produced a report that showed, among other things, that the introduction of binary logic would enable a machine of ENIAC's capability to be produced with only 6,000 valves instead of 18,000. This philosophy was seized upon, and the first of many binary digital computers, the EDSAC 1, was produced at Cambridge University. It is important to emphasise in this context that binary is purely an engineering expedient; it reduces the amount of equipment required and, hence, its universality in computer design and manufacture. There is no need for it to be the impenetrable barrier to understanding which it is in so many explanations. Binary is rather like tappets in a motor-car engine: vital to its proper and efficient functioning, but not something that need worry the user of the machine should he not know what they are.

Early in the 1950s the manufacturers plucked up sufficient courage to produce the so-called 'first-generation' computers. Like ENIAC, they were based on thermionic valves and, despite the application of the Princeton philosophy, were bulky, expensive and unreliable. Nevertheless, they accomplished prodigious feats of calculation when they were working, and thus found ready acceptance in university departments, research and development laboratories, and such like, where despite their lack of reliability, they provided useful results quickly, as well as providing useful operating experience for both programmers and engineers. With the commercial introduction of the transistor (to replace the thermionic valve, thus reducing volume and heat dissipation by an order of magnitude) the so-called 'second-generation' computers emerged about 1959–60, although Shockley had first invented the transistor in 1948. These were much more reliable (about 90 per cent) from the start, as well as being easier to operate. Moreover, they were up to one-hundred times faster than the first-generation machines, and since they cost about the same, they were, in effect, up to one hundred times cheaper. All these factors contributed to computers leaving the cossetted environment of universities and finding a place in commerce and industry. There was an increasing awareness that computers could be used for purposes other than calculation, and an awareness of their so-called 'data-processing' capability, although few recognised that this extended beyond routine matters such as payroll and accounting procedures. With the greatly enlarged capacity of the second-generation computers (due to their faster speed), coupled with improved engineering techniques for storage ('ferrite core store' and magnetic tape systems were introduced), more advanced programming techniques were developed, the main feature of these being that the user prepared his program in a 'high-level' computer language, which the computer itself translated into its own basic machine language. These languages are discussed more fully in Appendix 1.

As many different types of organisation (banks, insurance companies, refining industries, aviation, and so on) took advantage of the changed economics of computer power, the computer manufacturers were faced with the difficulty of providing suitable data-processing configurations for each type of application. They found themselves involved in special design problems to meet each particular requirement, and this was not conducive to economic production, reliability, or servicing; nor was it compatible with enabling systems to be enlarged as increasing uses were found for them. Most of these problems were overcome with the introduction of the so-called 'third-generation' computers in 1965-66, whose main feature was their modularity. Every system, requires a central processor, that is, the central store and control unit, but beyond that different users require different types of input/output devices (tape readers, card readers, analogue-to-digital converters, teleprinters, line printers, graph-plotters) and different combinations of 'file' stores (magnetic tape units, magnetic disc units, magnetic drum units). Thus, compatible units to provide a large variety of system configurations were highly desirable, and this is what the third-generation machines were largely able to provide.

TIME SHARING SYSTEMS

Accompanying the third-generation computers, however, there was a further increase in speed, some being capable of operating at a million basic operations a second, that is, a thousand times faster than the original ENIAC. This speed provides a new and remarkable opportunity: whereas ENIAC and the first-generation computers could perform a thousand operations a second for only one user at a time, a fast third-generation computer can, in principle, provide one thousand operations a second for up to one thousand users. This is the essence of what is called 'time-sharing', and it marked a significant new development in the application and distribution of computer power. Although the intrinsic difficulties of designing successful time-sharing systems are considerable, their use is now commonplace.

Time-sharing has the advantage of enabling the user to interface *directly* with the computer (albeit at a remote terminal), an advantage the pioneer user will recall, but one that was steadily withdrawn during the 1950s. The practice of the early days (late 1940s–early 1950s) by which a user took his own data and program to the computer, pressed the buttons, examined results, made changes, re-ran the program, and so on, until he obtained a satisfactory result had perforce to be abandoned in the name of efficiency. Fast computers, such as those of the second-generation, were economic only if the central processor was working almost continuously, and it could not do this while a user was pondering his program and deciding what to do next. The first change was to prevent users operating their own programs. This job was taken over by a computer operator who, because he was doing nothing else, became reasonably efficient at computer operation; also, because the operator knew nothing about the details of the program being operated, there was no tendency for him to interfere with the 'run'. As soon as a program stopped, it was returned to the user either with the completed results, where the program had worked satisfactorily, or with 'diagnostic' information about why it had stopped (automatically supplied by the computer) if the run was not completed. Even this method of working, however, involved the manual initiation by the computer operator of each separate program, during which time the expensive central processor was unproductive. This led to a further change, to 'batch-processing' on the more expensive computer installations. In this method of working, jobs are loaded into batches on magnetic tape (sometimes using a relatively less expensive auxiliary computer for the purpose), and a large part of the computer operator's job is taken over by a 'supervisor' or 'monitor' program which sequences the jobs through the computer with a minimum of delay. The results are commonly left on magnetic tapes (thus avoiding relatively slow on-line printing which ties up the central processor), which are then detached to operate an off-line printer. Although this greatly increases the 'throughput' of the computer, and thereby cheapens the cost of data-processing, a user may discover an inadvertent or trivial error in his program a day or so *after* he has delivered it to the computer office. This disadvantage may significantly lengthen the time taken to test out ('de-bug' is the term most frequently used) a new program, and discourage the use of the computer for smaller jobs.

Time-sharing, in effect, restores the operating console of the computer to the user, who by means of data-terminals can operate the computer *as if he were the only one using the machine.* How this is achieved in essence can be gleaned from considering the following. Suppose, hypothetically, that a particular user is typing data and/or instructions into a computer, via his local and immediately accessible data-terminal, at the impossibly high rate of ten keypresses a second; even this typing virtuosity would still leave some 100,000 millionths of a second between each keypress. Time, that is, for the computer to inspect the keyboard of every other user, and with time to spare in each second to do a little work on each user's program.* Yet to each user, typing as fast as he can, it still seems that the computer is working only for him. It is in this manner that a very fast computer can be made to perform many programs apparently simultaneously.

A time-sharing computer system must contain within itself some elaborate arrangement (usually called a 'supervisor' or 'monitor' program) for switching its facilities to and from each user in a rapid sequence that sensibly meets each user's requirements. Easily enough said, but 'each user's requirements' can vary so widely that any simple solution, however ingenious, could be seriously deficient in particular cases. 'Response time' will be an overriding consideration for a doctor or stockbroker requesting information about his patient or client, as it will be for the customer of an air-line seat reservation system. But for other users, efficient data-processing, implying high utilisation of expensive parts of the computer system, will be the over-riding consideration. Some users will require 'talk-back' interaction with the computer; others will wish to initiate only particular programs and get the results as quickly and cheaply as possible—but quickly and cheaply are conflicting criteria. All users will want a high standard of reliability and varying degrees of security for their 'files' and programs.

Satisfying these multiple-user considerations and a host of

---

*In fact, because a computer has only to inspect each keyboard to see if a character has been typed—a matter of a few millionths of a second per keyboard—rather than wait while it is being typed, then much more time than 100,000 millionths of a second is available between each keypress.

others, in sequencing input, output and storage devices, in preventing one program interfering with another, in providing translation from several computer languages, in encoding data for safe transmission, often over long distances (including satellites), and in logging times for charging purposes, and so on, present the designers with formidable problems. A number of commercial time-sharing systems are installed and working. The overall target is to divorce the user from the intracacies of input, output and storage devices between which the computer must continuously switch, in the same way that the telephone user is divorced from the complex switching processes that connect him from A to B. If, as is hoped, users with data terminals are to include not only doctors, nurses, technicians and administrators, but also housewives for shopping purposes, husbands for income-tax and carpentry calculations, and children for homework and instructional purposes, then it must become possible for users to have sufficient 'page-addressable' data storage (without the complications of cores, drums, discs and tapes) for them to make data transactions in an easily understandable language. The view of many computer experts is that this target is attainable and that considerable progress will be made towards attaining it within the next ten years or so. The sceptical reader may ponder the fact that it was only 15 years ago that the first reasonably reliable, reasonably priced, and reasonably operable computers (the second-generation) became available, and less than 15 years (1961) since the first astronaut orbited the earth.

The stage now emerging, in fact, is that of the 'computer utility' in which users with data-terminals may meter computer power in much the same way that they already meter electrical power or telephone time. As with early electric power stations and telephone exchanges, the numbers of users of computer power stations are still small. But national and even international grid or network systems are being thought of and are already being worked out for government organisations, for banking operations, and for airline bookings. Such developments will be greatly accelerated by the advent of global satellite communications.

SMALL COMPUTERS OR MINICOMPUTERS

Technical developments such as the transistor, the integrated circuit (IC) and now large-scale integration (LSI) have resulted in a steady 'micro-miniaturisation' of the computer until we now have commercially used processors and stores the size of small filing cabinets. Wherever electronic circuitry is involved the development has been along the lines of reduction in size and cost and increase in speed of performance. Peripherals have also shown a reduction in cost, although to a far less-marked extent.

This combination means that today's small computer systems are not only faster and smaller but are likely to be more cost-effective in many health-care applications than the large computers they will replace.

Since this trend is here to stay, it is worthwhile to review briefly the relative merits of large and small computer systems. Most jobs offered to a computer are of a trivial nature and are heavily related to the 'inputting' and 'outputting' of data, which tends to favour small computers. On the other hand, long runs, 'number crunching'* and file handling are better performed on large machines.

Initial costs are high with large machines and it is doubtful if the full capacity can be used until a long time after installation. The small computer can be expanded as need arises; the system is likely to be fully utilised all the time.

Response to interrupts (a signal from an instrument or from a patient monitoring transducer) is quicker on the small machine. The large machine is like a brontosaurus in this respect: stick a pin in the tail and minutes afterwards the head begins to turn!

A small computer is more easily 'configured' and 'reconfigured'. This means that the system can be put together in some different way much more easily. Individual modules are more cheaply updated and replaced.

A large computer system needs a special environment, false floor to cover wiring, special air conditioning, and so forth, while the small computer system needs only an office environment.

These special computer rooms too easily soon develop into inviolable, holy sanctums where only technical staff may tread. They create a barrier between the eventual user (nurse, clinician or administrator) and the computer staff. And they are very expensive. Given small computers, more clinicians and nurses are

*The common jargon for repetitive arithmetical calculations.

likely to approach the machine and become involved by obtaining actual experience of using the system.

Too often, operating programs have been developed by the hardware manufacturer with only hardware and system efficiency in mind. Too little account has been taken of the user and his interests. It has been necessary to introduce into the user's organisation all manner of computer orientated staff who have no experience or knowledge of the user's business or procedures. A steadily increasing specialist interface has been built up, which has invariably resulted in a communication block and unrealistic and ineffective use of the computer. The computer system has not been integrated in the organisation and has been run largely for the benefit of the computer staff.

As we shall see in a later chapter, many medical applications of computers are naturally more suited to small computers, such as patient or instrument monitoring. Specific applications are always likely to be better performed on small dedicated machines. It has been too readily accepted that in medical record handling and in total hospital information systems a large processor is essential.

Large computing systems often have the developed programs and procedures so necessary to such systems. However, as mini-computers develop sophisticated software,* it becomes feasible to try distributed or multi-processor solutions. These will allow experts in particular areas to develop their own systems and eventually to integrate these sub-systems into a total hospital system. What seems most likely is that hospital systems will be combinations of small and large machines. The satellite terminal is an example of the combination of the two, allowing computer power to be distributed over a wide area. Closely integrated networks of computers are the likely pattern of the future.

NON-DIGITAL COMPUTERS IN MEDICINE

Analogue computers have limited application in medical automation, so they will be referred to only briefly. They are so called because they represent a physical analogy of formulae, which in an idealised way may effectively characterise, or form a useful model of certain situations as, for example, in cardiopulmonary

*The jargon for written instructions; programs, procedures and so on.

analysis. The low accuracy of analogue computers limits the complexity of the models employed, but this can be overcome by using 'hybrid' computers, in which certain elements (e.g. integrators) function digitally to preserve accuracy. On the few occasions where analogue computers suffice, they are probably the cheapest, quickest and most effective way of dealing with a problem.

Other examples of specialised computers used in medicine are the frequency analyser, auto-correlator and cross-correlator, and the response averager. A detailed technical description would be out of context here, but it is sufficient to note that each type of machine embodies a particular analytical method in its physical construction (i.e. it is a physical analogue of a particular data-procedure), and that the four analytical methods mentioned have been used commonly in the study of electrical signals of physiological origin (e.g. electrocardiogram and electroencephalogram). A common problem with such signals is that the desired information is often obscured by other signals (e.g. fetal by maternal electrocardiogram), or by background (electrical) 'noise'. All these methods provide useful ways of increasing the signal-to-noise ratio.

Before the advent of the digital computer, it was necessary to have recourse to a special-purpose machine for each analytical method (i.e. each calculation), but with the general-purpose small computers now available the role of the special-purpose machine is likely to become even more limited.

4
The Features of a Data Processing System

REPLACING MEANING BY STRUCTURE: PROGRAMMING AND
DATA PREPARATION

BEING A MACHINE, a computer cannot accept data in any form; certainly not in the form in which it is commonly kept in paper filing systems. Unlike the cerebral cortex, the computer, being a machine, has no ability to interpret *meaning*, which must perforce be replaced by something else. In practice it is replaced by structure. Data must be set down *systematically* according to some format or other, so that similar items appear in similar positions; e.g. age, sex, address, and so on, should appear in the same position on each separate document. If this were not so, that is, if the designer of the computer procedure could not assume a common structure to the data contained on separate documents, then his procedure would have to incorporate an additional feature to identify each particular item. This is not impossible, but it does mean additional complication, and is wasteful. For these reasons it is avoided wherever possible. Apart from each item being assigned to a particular position, or sequence, on the original documents, each item must be limited to a code number, or a specified vocabulary, or a specified length (called a 'field'). These problems are discussed at length later, but in essence *the data must conform to some agreed specification, to which the designer of the computer procedure (or program) can work.* Almost any specification could be acceptable, but both economy and simplicity in designing the computer procedure will result from adopting the simplest form of data that is acceptable to the user. This last point is often the over-riding consideration; otherwise there can be no universal rules, since data arise in different forms: a bank cheque has little in common with a medical record or a radiograph or an ECG.

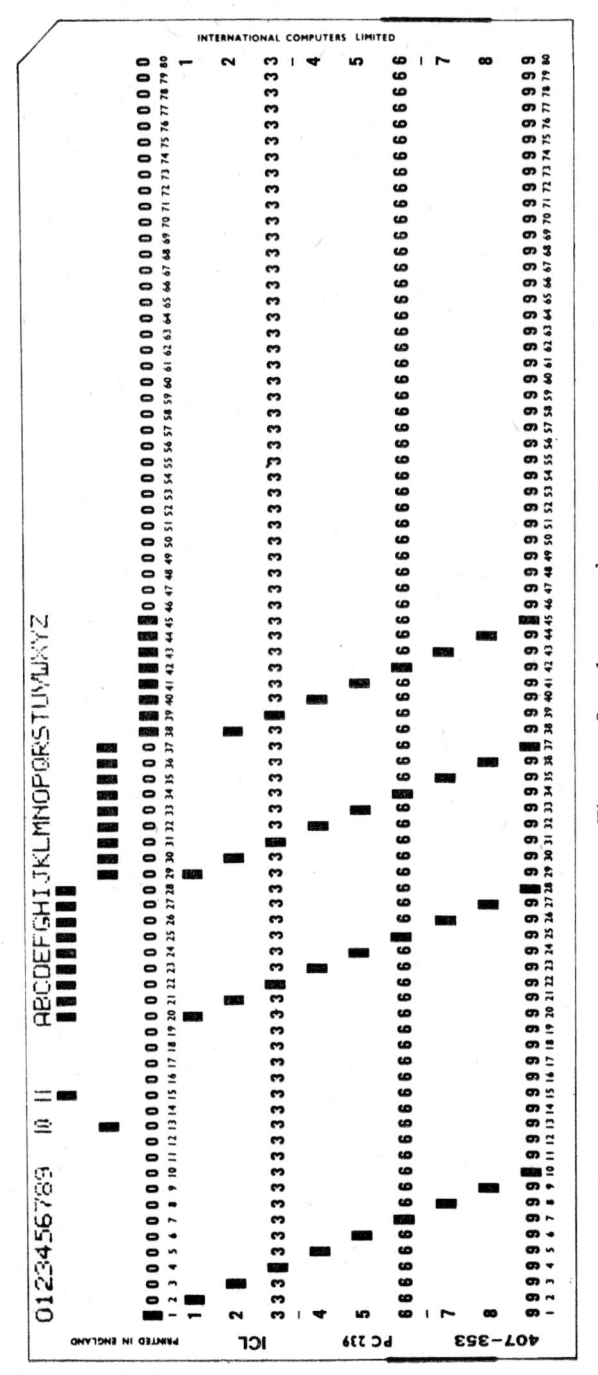

Figure 1. 80-column card

Secondly, data must be digitally structured, in order that they can be inserted in a computer. The reasons for this are discussed later. The most common way of inserting data in a digitally structured form into a computer is either on punch cards or paper tape (other newer ways are discussed later). At the time of writing, more than 99 per cent of all data is entered into computers in this way and will be so for many years to come. Where data originate in the form of handwritten or typewritten documents, as is the case of medical records, the transfer process is as illustrated in Plate 1A. Data sheets are handed to a punch operator who types out the information on a key-board with a punch attachment. As each key (numeral, letter, space, and so on) is depressed, it produces either a coded row of holes in a length of paper tape or a column of holes in a punched-card, thus converting a batch of documents into either a continuous length of paper tape or a batch of punched cards. Specimens of punched paper tape and punched cards are shown in Plate 1B and Figure 1, and Plates 1C and 2A show equipments for producing punched paper tape and punched cards.

When data originate from instruments such as an electro-cardiograph, an encephalograph, a blood pressure recorder, or an auto-analyser, however, a different technique is required to structure the data digitally. An analyser actually provides an electric voltage in an analogue form. This is converted into digital form by a device known as an Analogue-to-Digital converter (ADC). This device is simply a means of electrically conditioning a signal from an instrument so that it can be accepted by the digital computer system. The system will be programmed to calibrate and correct a series of signals into a reading which can be output on paper tape, line printer, and so on. It is sometimes necessary when the signal rate is very high to collect all raw output from the instrument onto magnetic tape or disc to be analysed later.

Two-dimensional data, or pictures such as radiographs, may also be digitally structured for insertion into a computer. In this case a further piece of equipment called a *flying-spot scanner* needs to be interposed between the picture instrument (e.g. X-ray machine) and the analogue-to-digital converter. The flying spot-scanner consists of an electric flying spot which scans the picture a line-at-a-time (television-wise) at something like 200 lines to the inch. Each spot in each line is coded by the analogue-to-digital converter into a contrast level and the code for each spot is either punched on paper-tape, or more speedily recorded on magnetic tape. In this way a picture is turned into a continuous length of punched paper tape, or of digital magnetic tape or onto a disc.

PROGRAMMING

So much for data. Preparing a procedure or program for insertion into a computer is rather more complicated. Being a machine, the computer cannot accept a procedure stated in ordinary everyday language. Unlike the human brain, which can understand a variety of idioms, dialects, and vocabularies in a variety of syntactical combinations, a computer cannot; it can only accept procedures which (a) have been structured systematically, and (b) coded into one or other of the many so-called 'computer languages' of which COBOL, FORTRAN, CORAL and ALGOL* are the best known and most frequently used at the present time.

To see what is involved in some detail let us consider a hypothetical situation, which nevertheless exemplifies the basic thinking behind all computerised medical records procedures. An institution, let us suppose, reviews the salary of each of its 1,000 employees on their respective birthdays, so that each and every day 1,000 records must be scanned to identify those with birthdays. The problem is how to 'systemise' this procedure so that a machine could carry it out. The solution, once the knack of looking at the world through data-processing spectacles has been acquired, is simple:—

(a) *store* all the 1,000 records in the computer;
(b) *insert* the current date;
(c) *subtract* the day and month part of the current date from the day and month part of each date of birth, in turn;
(d) *print out* the names of those for which the answer is zero.

Essentially, therefore, the procedure consists of a thousand subtractions, and a thousand 'zero-or-not' decisions. Just the sort of thing a computer can do, and do incredibly quickly; in fact, a computer can perform as many as one million subtractions a

See **Glossary**

38   Medical Automation

second so that the above procedure would occupy the computer for less than a second a day. Elaboration can be built on this simple theme: to determine which of those with birthdays are also male, a similar device is employed. Assuming that male and female are denoted as such by the letters M and F, then all that is necessary is that M be 'subtracted' from the sex data of each record to see if the result is zero or not. M-M will be zero,

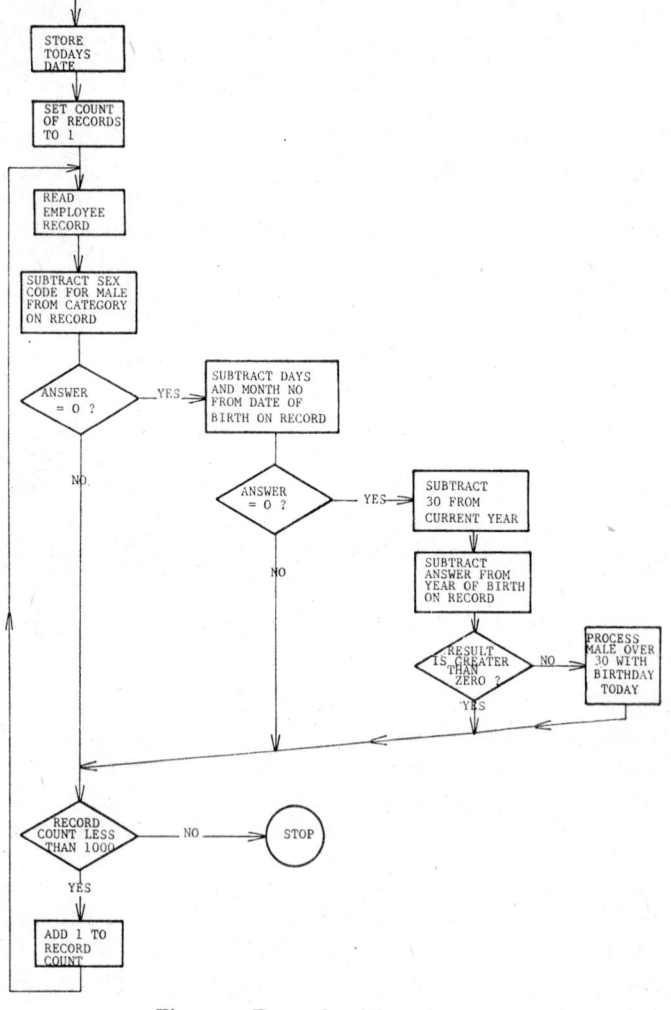

Figure 2. Example of flow chart

while F-M is not. The point is that computers can just as readily store alphabetical data as numerical data, and they can 'subtract' one item (number or word) from another. Subtraction and testing zero is thus a common device for determining whether a person's record contains a particular item. To select all those patients with measles, one simply 'subtracts' measles from the disease category in each record, printing out the patient names (or numbers) when the result is zero. In addition to discriminating between zero-or-not, a computer can also discriminate between positive-or-negative which enables 'more' or 'less' decisions to be made. For example, in the case of the 1,000 employees above, we may wish to ascertain which are more than 30 years of age. The device here is to subtract 30 from the current year, e.g. 69 − 30 = 39, and then subtract 39 from the employee's year of birth; if the result is positive he is less than 30, whereas if the result is negative he is over 30. Figure 2 shows how such sequences of increasing complexity can be built up and 'flow-charted'. All the machine operators are set out in capital letters, and it will be noticed that to extract records with multiple attributes requires only SUBTRACTION, TRANSFER, REPEAT, ZERO-OR-NOT TEST, and POSITIVE-OR-NEGATIVE TEST. The rest is tedious organisation, which no one would be disposed to embark on but for the fact that each of these basic operations takes only about a millionth of a second to be performed. The business of analysing a task into an organised sequence of basic machine operations is part of what is called 'programming'. Once this is done it is a relatively straightforward process to 'code' this organised sequence into an acceptable 'computer language', the most basic of which is 'machine code', more advanced forms of which are 'high level languages' (COBOL, FORTRAN, CORAL, ALGOL*).

Preparing a data-procedure for a computer thus requires—

(a) a method or system to deal with the problem;
(b) flow-charting a step-by-step sequence of basic operations;
(c) coding into a computer language;
(d) conversion into punched paper tape or punched cards.

The whole activity is known as *programming*, those who carry it out are known as *programmers*, and the result (a data-procedure set out in a language acceptable to a computer) is called a *program*.

*See Glossary

Not all programmers are capable of the whole task. Junior programmers will concentrate mainly on coding, and graduate to flow-charting; many will stay at this level. The more able and creative will concentrate on the problem-solving area of determining methods or systems. This latter requires more than computer skill; it requires, in addition, a detailed technical knowledge of the problem itself. Numerical analysts will be best suited to finding methods of solution to mathematical problems; but business systems analysts assisted by O & M and OR specialists will be best suited to business problems; whereas medical systems analysts, musical systems analysts, traffic systems analysts, will be best suited to their respective fields.

The role of the systems analysts and programmers in the design of data-processing is analogous to the relationship between architects and builders. The systems analyst, like the architect, must in the first instance *determine the main objectives of the user*, which may be to increase the productivity of laboratories, to increase the effectiveness of diagnostic procedures, or to increase the level of immunity in a given community. He will then structure and enumerate the relevant data-procedures that are necessary, and will produce their specifications and priorities. At this point he engages the attention of the chief programmer, the builder, so that part of their common ground will be discussion on methods of solution. Once agreed between them, the chief programmer and his team have a fairly closely defined job of work to create respective programs according to the agreed specifications.

Systems analysis then, specifies what data and data-procedures are required to meet overall objectives. Programming translates these respectively into data formats and working computer programs which meet the systems analysts' specifications. Such is the main division of the overall responsibility. From the point of view of the computer, however, it means that a number of data-procedures have to be carried out, for each of which both the data and the procedure have been converted into either lengths of punched paper tape or stacks of punched cards.

A GENERAL-PURPOSE DATA-PROCESSING SYSTEM

The basic configuration of any computer system consists (Figure 3) of a store, an input device and an output device, and a control

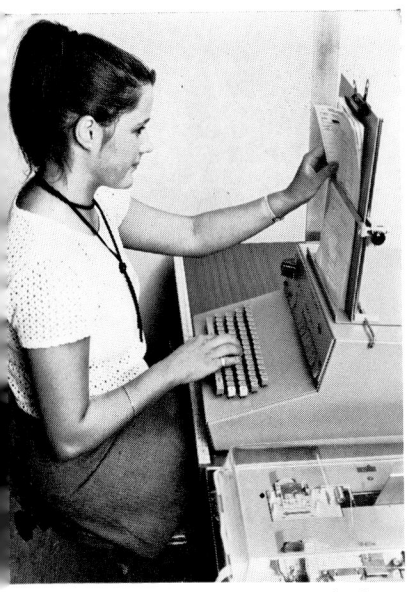

A Transferring data sheets to punched form (Courtesy *Computer Weekly*)

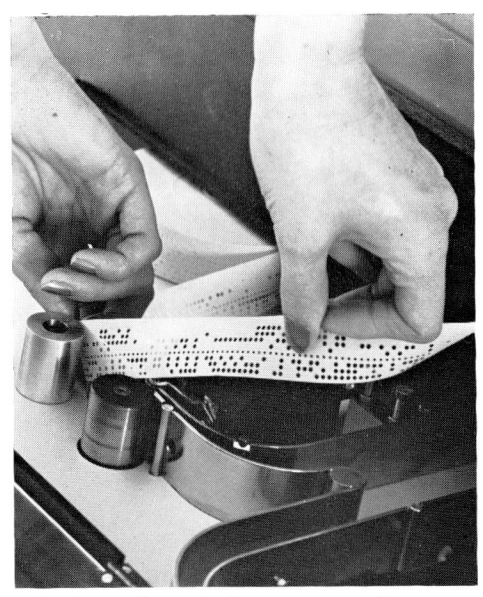

B A piece of punched paper tape (Courtesy Peter Waugh)

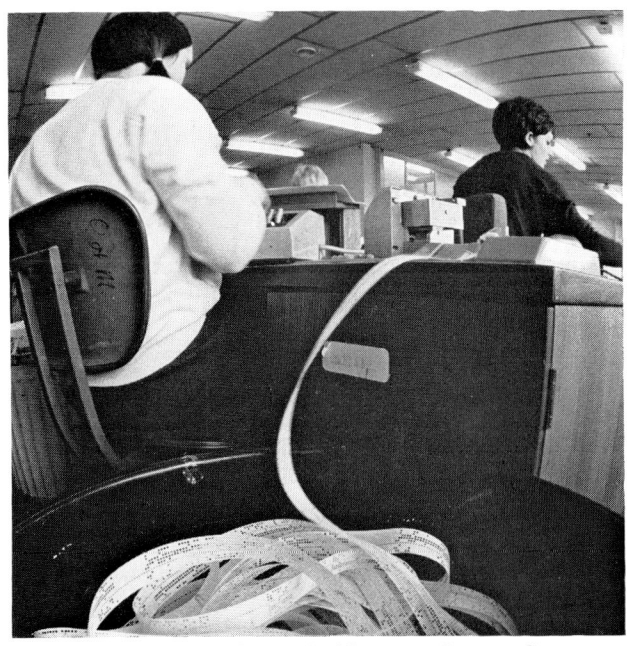

C Paper tape keyboard punch (Courtesy Sanaco Computer Services)

PLATE I

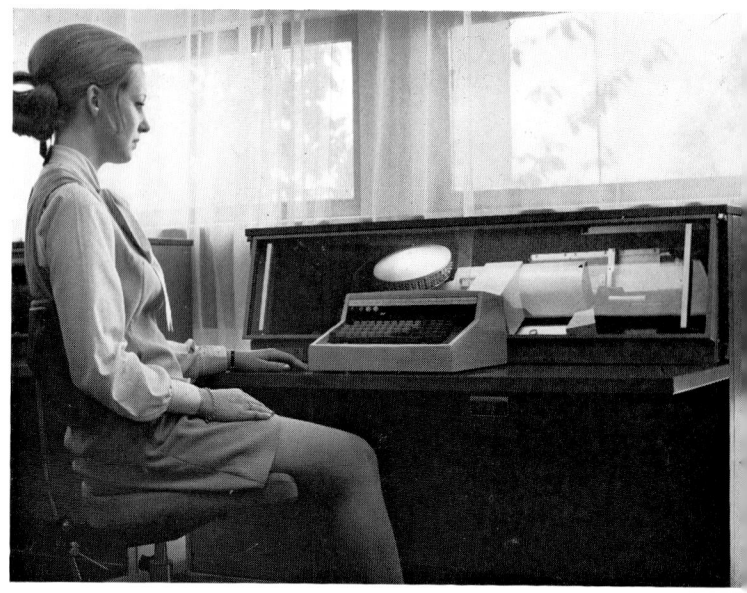

A A punched card keyboard punch (Courtesy International Computers Ltd)

B A paper tape reader (Courtesy International Computers Ltd)

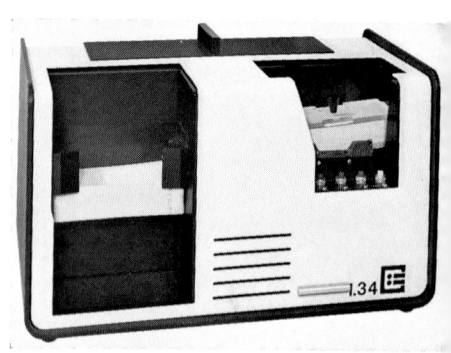

C A card reader (Courtesy Computer Technology Ltd)

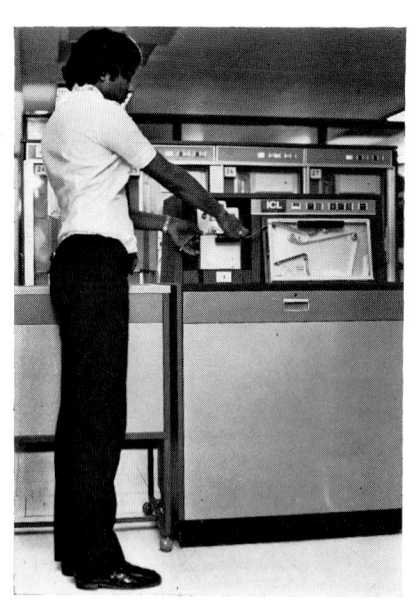

PLATE 2

A Magnetic ink character reader (Courtesy International Computers Ltd)

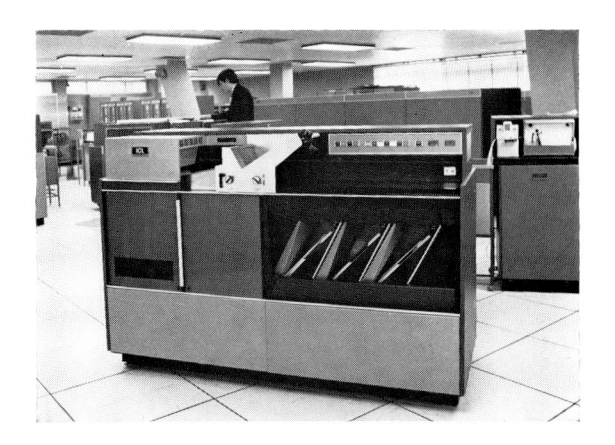

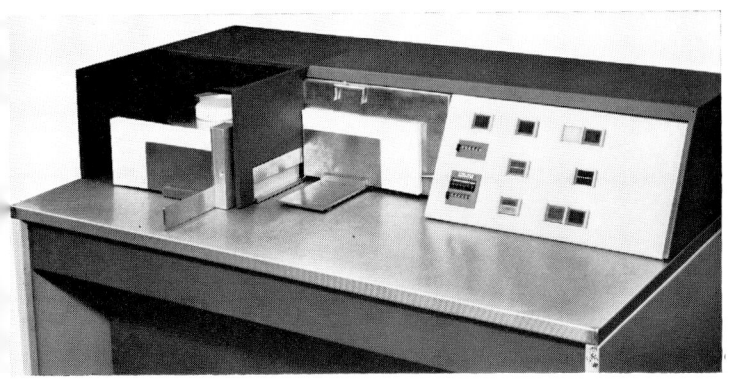

B Optical character reader (Courtesy *Computer Weekly*)

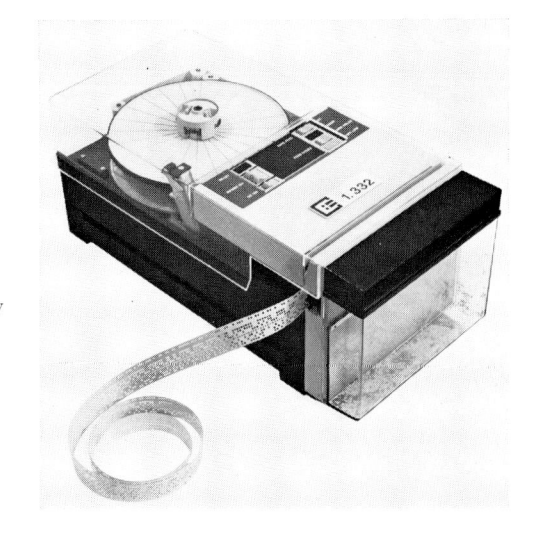

C Paper tape punch (Courtesy Computer Technology Ltd)

PLATE 3

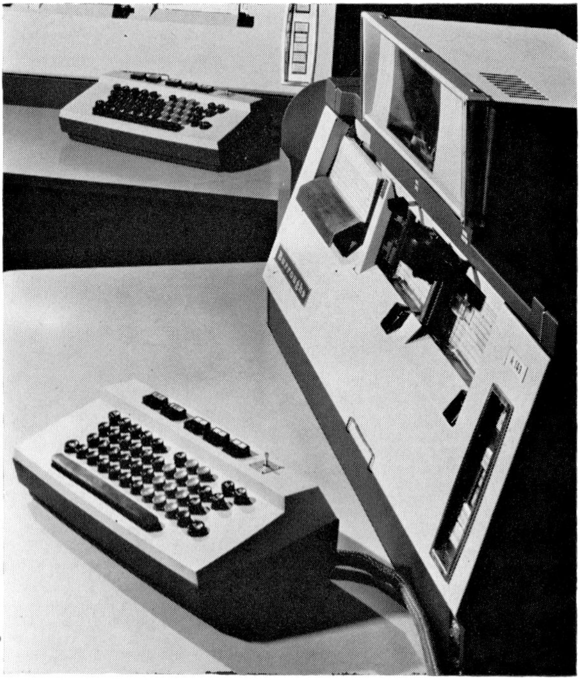

A Card punch (Courtesy Burroughs)

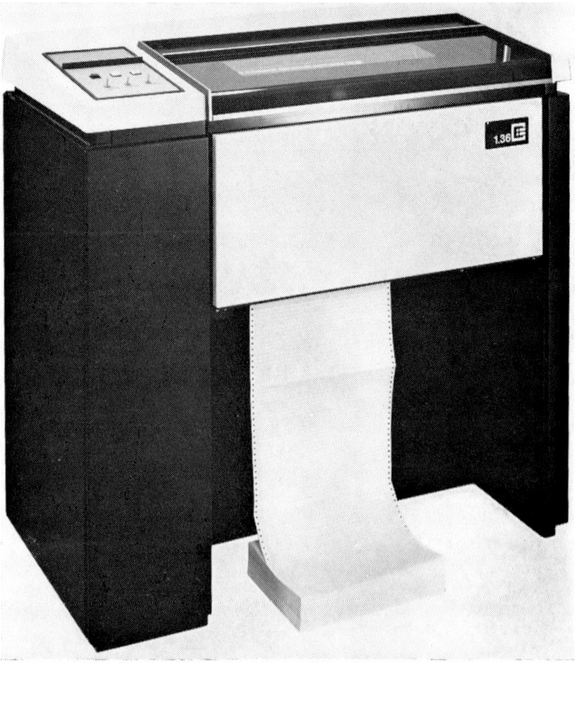

B Line printer (Courtesy Computer Technology I

PLATE 4

mechanism. The program tape is inserted into the input device, and at the press of a button, is transferred to the store; then the data is similarly transferred to the store. At the press of the start button the control unit causes the programmed procedure to operate on the data, and results are presented via the output device, which may be an automatic typewriter. Because the store in which these operations take place is fairly expensive, as one might expect of a device operating at a million operations a second, it is usual to provide less expensive 'back up' or 'file' storage in the form of magnetic tape units, magnetic disc units,

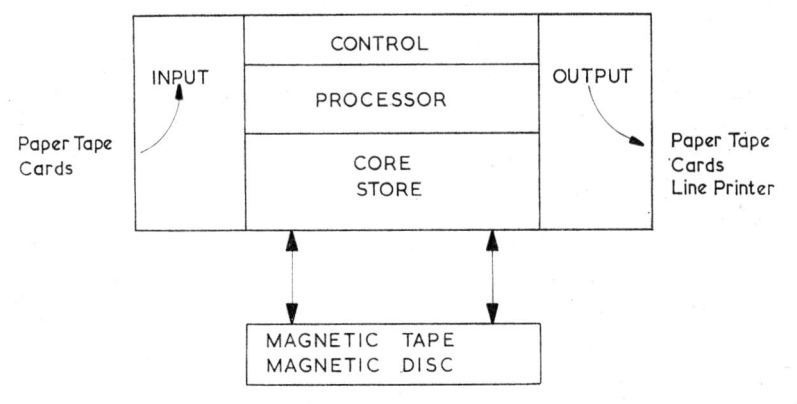

Figure 3. Basic plan of computer

or magnetic drum units, for filing records, directories, programs, and so on.

Because data arise in a variety of ways and can be digitally structured in a variety of ways for insertion into the computer, it is common to find different kinds of input devices connected to a computer. Similarly, a number of different output devices attempt to provide results from the computer in a form best suited to a particular user's needs. A typical general-purpose 'data-processing system' is illustrated in Figure 4. At the heart of it is the 'central processor', as it is called, the combination of store and control in which all data-procedures are actually carried out; the Americans call it the 'main frame'. The rest are the so-called peripheral units, or simply 'peripherals', which consist of various input devices, various output devices, and various large-capacity storage devices. It is unlikely that any particular data-processing

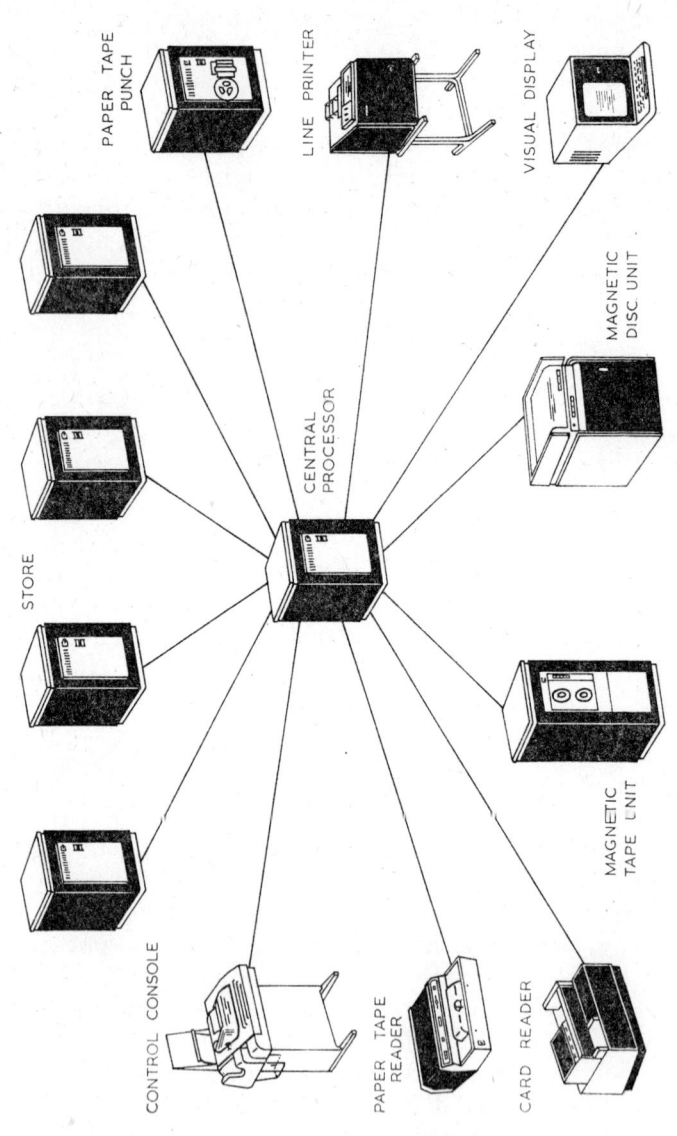

Figure 4. General-purpose data processing system

system will contain every particular kind of input, output and storage device. It will very much depend on the uses to which the data-processing system is to be put, and one of the difficult initial decisions every purchaser must make, advised by his systems analysts, is what particular configuration will best suit his particular purposes. Some of the more salient features of the most commonly encountered input and output devices are as follows.

INPUT DEVICES

Punched Paper Tape Reader and Punched Card Reader

These devices respectively transfer punched paper tape data and punched card data into the computer. They operate essentially by shining a narrow beam of light across each row of holes, in the case of punched paper tape, and across each column of holes, in the case of punch cards. The patterns of holes and non-holes are then converted by photo-electric cells into a corresponding pattern of electric pulses, in which form they can be electronically dealt with. At the time of writing more than 99 per cent of all data is entered into computers via tape or card readers, and although this is likely to change in the next decade, they are still likely to be the most commonly used input devices for many years to come (Plate 2B and C).

Magnetic Ink Character Reader (MICR)

The business of converting data to punched form in order to insert it in a computer is tedious, time-consuming, error-prone and, of course, it costs money. The incentive therefore has always existed to produce a device that could 'read' data directly. Unfortunately, there are so many styles of print, so many different typewriter type faces, so many different sizes and textures of paper, so many different styles of handwriting that designers have long since excluded the practical possibility of a universal character reader. This is not to say, however, that they have not been without success in designing character readers, but the problem has been the exacting one of reliability. Even a 99·9 per cent reliability means one wrong character in every 1,000 and this is an unacceptable error rate, so most approaches have concentrated on designing special styles of typeface which can be read reliably, and by far the most successful of these to date has been the magnetic ink character typeface, which is to be seen on most bank cheques. Each character produces a sufficiently different magnetic field from any other character that it can be reliably and accurately sensed at speed. To each separate character the MICR device assigns a unique code of electric pulses, similar to that assigned by the punched paper tape and punched card readers (Plate 3A).

Optical Character Reader (OCR)

This is very similar in principle to the MICR device, the essential difference being that a special typeface is used to produce a sufficiently different distribution of ink for each character (under practical conditions of smudge, dirt and so on), that can be photo-electrically sensed, and, hence, unequivocally assigned a unique code of electric pulses. Except in banking, where MICR is widely used, character readers have as yet a limited use, but now that reliable equipment is being produced, their use is likely to increase (Plate 3B).

Mark Sensing

This is a technique that pre-dates computers, and that relies on the fact that particular *positions* on a document represent particular characters. By scanning each position and sensing the presence or absence of marks (usually by photo-electric means), the marked characters can be assigned an appropriate code of electric pulses. The technique requires, of course, that all possible, or allowable, answers are already laid out on the document, and a set of marks determines a particular selection. It has considerable advantages in particular situations such as many types of survey, but in situations where a great variety of answers has to be allowed for it can require some very unwieldy documents, and for this reason its use is limited.

Analogue-to-Digital Converter

This device is for inputting continuous signals such as those generated by instruments. The instrument is sampled at frequent intervals, and each sample is assigned a unique code of electric pulses. It has been more fully described previously in this chapter (page 36).

Remote Typewriter/Teleprinter

This device operates in a very similar way to a keyboard punch. The essential feature is that each keypress corresponding to a particular symbol activates a set of solenoids which generate a coded set of electric pulses for transmission to the computer.

It can thus be seen that there is a variety of ways of inserting data into a computer. Each has particular characteristics, but, in general, punched card readers and punched paper tape readers are most commonly used. Every input device has the effect of transforming data into coded arrays of electrical pulses, which is the only way in which data can be dealt with by an electronic digital computer.

OUTPUT DEVICES

Automatic Typewriter/Teleprinter

Results from a computer are produced in sequence, one character at a time, each character being in the form of an array of electric pulses. Each array activates a selection of solenoids which, in turn, activate a particular key of the keyboard. The mechanical working of keyboards limits printing speeds to tens of characters per second. The arrays of electric pulses can in fact be transmitted over wire (commonly via the telephone/teleprinter networks) to activate remotely placed printers.

Tape Punch and Card Punch

Each array is used to activate a selection of solenoids which, in turn, activate mechanical punches that produce a corresponding pattern of holes in each row of paper tape or in each column of a punched card. Punching speeds are limited to tens of characters per second (Plate 3C and 4A).

Line Printer

In situations involving a considerable amount of printing, such as producing thousands of gas-bills, printing one character at a time is far too slow. This is overcome in the line printer by using the arrays of, say, 100 or 200 characters to set up a whole line of type, which is then printed out at once. A typical line printer will print at a thousand lines a minute (Plate 4B).

Graph Plotter

With the advent of the computer the possibility, and with it the danger, exists of producing data at such a rate and in such a way (e.g. statistical tabulations) that there is too much to be assimilated. Intelligent use, therefore, requires a continuous examination to see for what purpose(s) the data are used, and whether any means of selection and presentation by the computer will facilitate its use. Presenting data graphically is one such means, hence the role of the automatic graph plotter. Programmed procedures can determine the form and manner of presentation, and if a graph is to be produced a suitable 'output program' will cause the computer to provide its results as a sequence of x and y co-ordinates. The automatic graph plotter is a device which will accept the x and y co-ordinates in the form of arrays of electric pulses from the computer and convert them into voltages for driving the pen to a particular position. A sequence of such co-ordinates then moves the pen to draw a corresponding graph (Plate 5A).

Activators

Where a computer is 'on-line', such as when directly connected to traffic sensing devices, or to cockpit instruments, or to patient monitoring instruments, the results from the computer are often required not in tabulated or graphical form, but in a form that can activate traffic signals, or switches, or light indicators. In this case the computer's results, coded in electrical pulses in the usual way, are transmitted by wire to activate remotely placed switches.

Visual Display Unit (VDU)

The visual display unit (Plate 5B) is a versatile input-output device. It combines a television-type screen with a typewriter-like keyboard. Data and programs can be typed into the computer from the keyboard, and information from the computer can be called up, virtually instantaneously, on the television-type tube. The basic principles are essentially the same as for other input-output devices: each keypress on the keyboard produces a coded array of electric pulses—the form in which a character can be entered into the computer. A group or sequence of characters can constitute a message which, under the control of a suitable programmed procedure, can initiate computer action. The action may, for example, take the form of a records search of the type outlined earlier in the section on programming, and the resultant findings can be displayed on the television-type tube. The way in which this latter aspect is achieved is as follows. A coded set of pulses from the computer for, say, the letter M is used to activate either a small program or some special circuitry which 'writes' the letter M on the television-type tube; and so on for every other character that is to be displayed. A further refinement exists in the form of a 'light pen' which enables the user to 'write' information—messages or drawings—directly onto the face of the television tube. How such messages, lines, curves and other symbols are dealt with by the computer will depend entirely on what computer procedures have been devised to work with them. For example, it is possible to write a rough sketch of a rectangle on the face of the television-type tube with the light pen, and then via a keyboard message, initiate a computer program that will draft out the rectangle so that it is exact dimensionally. Elaborations of this technique are the basis of 'computer graphics' or 'computer-aided design'. The many ramifications that are possible into computer-aided teaching, computer-aided editing, computer-aided typesetting, computer-aided recall of management and diagnostic information, are under active development in many centres throughout the world, and it is certain that we can look forward to a wide application of this technique. For what we are witnessing, in this context, is not the computer carrying out isolated single data-procedures, but a man-machine interaction in which stylised messages of increasing verisimilitude with ordinary conversation are exchanged between man and the computer. Designers, managers or researchers can ask the question 'what if', and the full implications, which might take man-months on paper, may be elicited at electronic speeds. Thus, with the introduction of the VDU the computer truly becomes an extension of brain function, without contradicting any of the cautions that have been presented earlier. It may thus be seen that there exists a variety of ways of 'outputting' data from a computer, each having particular merit in particular situations. Every output device has the effect of transforming data (presented one character at a time in sequence by the computer, in the form of coded electrical pulses) into a form that is assimilable by a human being; this may take the form of a printed record, a graph, a drawing, or a flashing light, and so on.

Data, as we have seen, may be entered into, and extracted from the central processor in a variety of ways, the essential reason for this variety being that the electronic arrangements of the central processor cannot deal directly with data in the form in which they naturally originate or are used. Each character must be inserted sequentially into the central processor as a coded array of electric pulses, and results are presented by the central processor one character at a time as a coded array of electrical pulses. Another limitation of the central processor derives from the fact that *it houses the store in which data are actively processed*, and 'active storage' is still relatively expensive (although getting less so). To store all data in this type of storage, whether active or not would be a costly operation and, not surprisingly therefore, engineers have developed much cheaper systems of 'file' or 'backing-up' storage for accommodating bulk data which are not being immediately processed by the computer. A description of the salient features of the principal file storage devices follows.

STORAGE DEVICES

Magnetic Tape Unit

This is still the most commonly used file store (Plate 6A). Essentially it consists of a reel of magnetic tape (very much like audio tape in appearance) about the size of a reel of cinematographic film. It is usually about 3,000 ft long, and characters are stored in rows, in a similar way in which they are stored on punched paper tape, the essential difference being that instead of holes and non-holes, they are stored as magnetic marks of two polarities. Whereas punched paper tape stores about ten characters to the inch, magnetic tape can store up to as many as one thousand characters to the inch, a typical tape in fact storing between 10 million and 100 million characters, depending on the type of tape and the packing density. This, of course, is a lot of information, especially when one remembers that it can be carried in a brief case, or kept in a desk drawer. To get a record onto magnetic tape, the record is usually first converted into punched paper tape or punched cards. Devices are, however, increasingly being introduced to key data straight onto magnetic tape. The record

A A graph plotter
(Courtesy International
Computers Ltd)

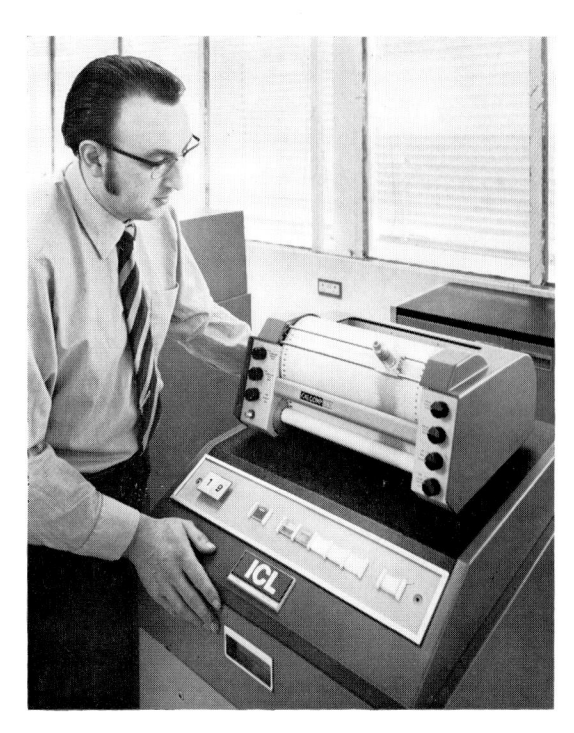

B A visual display unit
(Courtesy Burroughs)

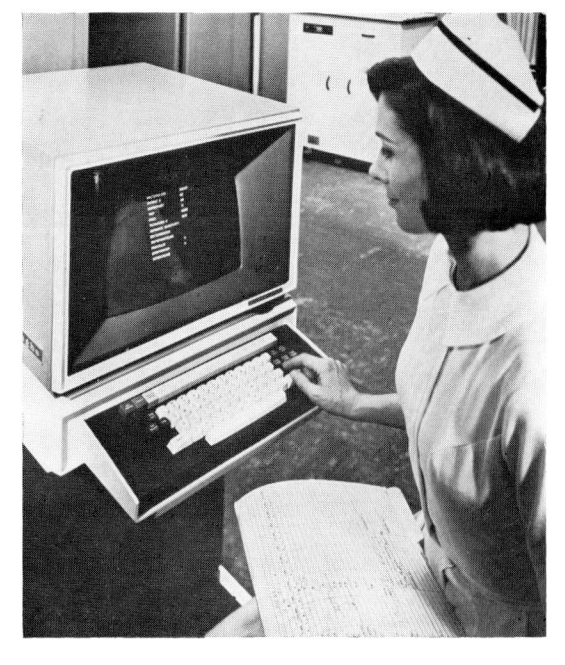

PLATE 5

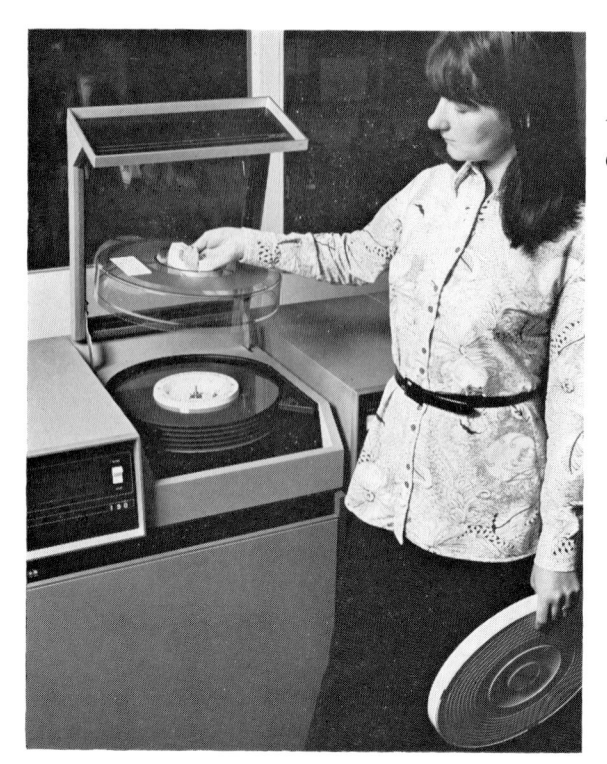

A Magnetic tape unit (Courtesy International Computers Ltd)

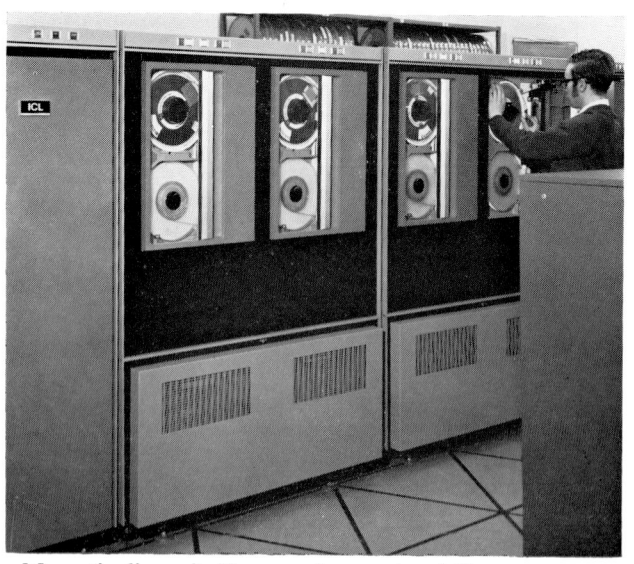

B Magnetic disc unit (Courtesy International Computers Ltd)

PLATE 6

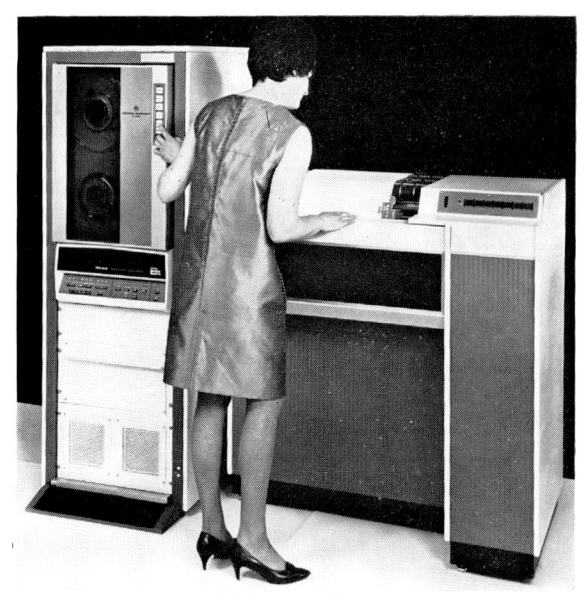

A Magnetic tape driving off-line printer (Courtesy Scientific Furnishings)

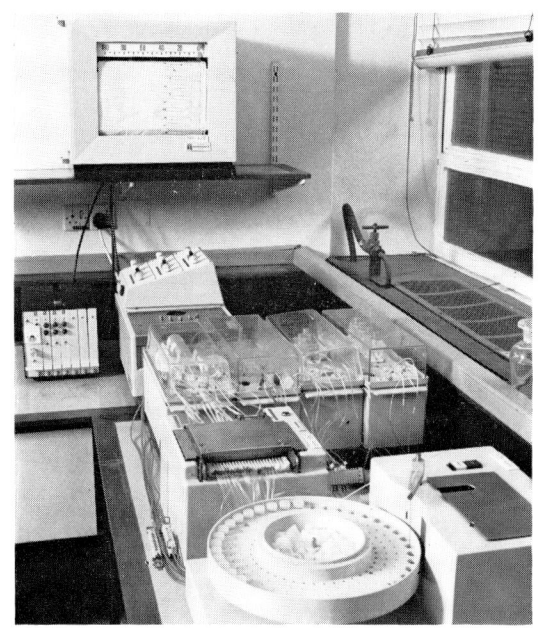

B View of Technicon Auto-Analyzer (Courtesy Computer Technology Ltd)

PLATE 7

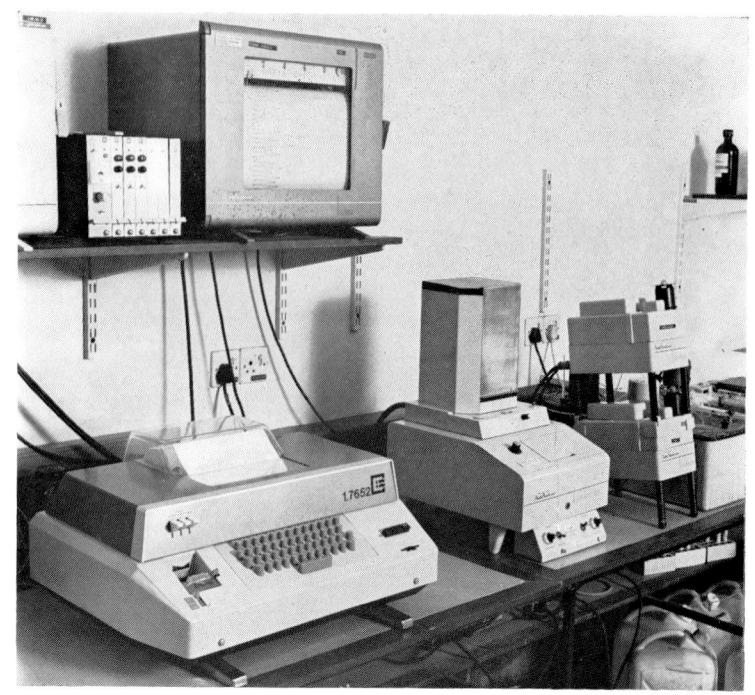

A Pen recorder and Auto-Analyzer (Courtesy Computer Technology Ltd)

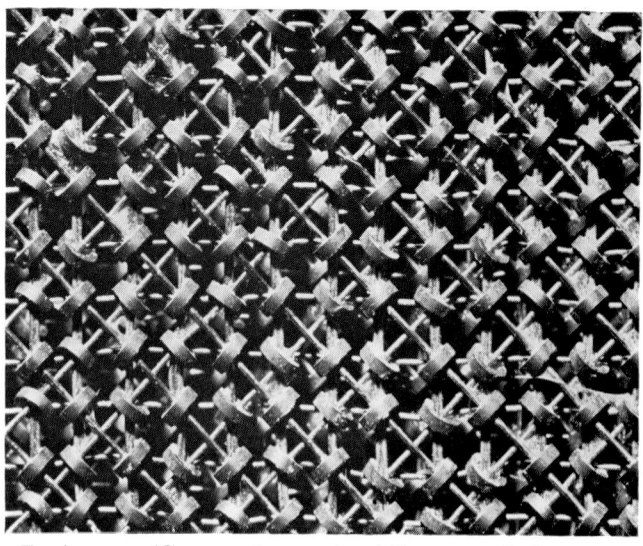

PLATE 8   B Ferrite cores (Courtesy International Computers Ltd)

in the punched form is then inserted into a punched paper tape reader or a card reader, as appropriate, and a reel of magnetic tape is attached to a magnetic tape handler. Then, when the start button of the computer is pressed, the central processor, operating a suitable 'input program', transfers each character from the reader, converts it into electric pulse form, and then uses these pulses to produce a corresponding magnetic pattern on the magnetic tape (Plate 6A). Data 'filed' in this way can then be kept in a safe place until required for 'processing'. Depending on the operations, whether those of an insurance company or a medical records system, a number of magnetic tape handlers may be connected to a central processor.

Magnetic Disc Unit

Owing to the fact that magnetic tape stores data serially along its length, those records nearer the end of its length will obviously take longer to access than those at the beginning; in the worst case several minutes may be required. For many applications this delay is not significant, but in those types of situation where one wishes to retrieve a particular record quickly—in particular when on-line data-terminals are used to summon a record—a delay of several minutes may be unacceptable. It is this problem that the magnetic disc unit has been designed to overcome. The way in which it works can be guessed at from its original name as a 'juke-box store'. It consists of a number of magnetic discs, rather like large gramophone records, about 20 to 30 inches in diameter. Data is stored (in character codes) in concentric circles on both sides of the discs, some six or so of which are fitted to a common axis (Plate 6B). It is rather like mounting half-a-dozen discs on a gramophone turntable. With independent 'recording/reading heads' which move radially across each side of each disc, data at any point in the disc unit can be 'accessed' very quickly. Since each concentric track stores about 4,000 characters, and since each side of each disc contains some 100 tracks, then the facility offered by a typical magnetic disc unit is that of retrieving data from any one of some 4 or 8 million characters (depending on the particular characteristics) in less than a tenth of a second. It has, therefore, better 'random access' than magnetic tape. Depending on requirements, a multiple number of magnetic disc units can be connected to a central processor.

Magnetic Drum Units

Magnetic drum units consist of a magnetically coated cylinder mounted on an axis along the length of the cylinder. Data is stored on parallel co-axial tracks around the surface of the cylinder, and each track has its own recording/reading head. Since the cylinder rotates at high speed the longest 'access time' for a particular item of data is the time it takes for the drum to rotate once about its access, usually some thousandths of a second. Magnetic drum units were the only file storage units available on computers, until the introduction of magnetic tape units in the late '50s, and magnetic disc units in recent years. They are less commonly used today, but since they have fast access times they are often used for storing programs which the processor can call down as required.

It can be seen, therefore, that there are many ways of providing 'file' storage, and by bringing together multiple numbers of the units described, enough flexibility exists to meet the requirements of almost any data-processing situation.

Although we have talked of all these peripheral units as being directly connected, i.e. on-line, to the central processor, this is not invariably the case. As already suggested, equipment now exists for typing data directly onto magnetic tapes to avoid the intermediate stages of punched media and transfer via the central processor; 'off-line' line printers (Plate 7A) and graph-plotters exist which may be loaded with either magnetic tapes or punched paper tapes and thus can operate independently and in separate locations from the central processor. The permutations are many, but enough has been said to range over the principal characteristics of general-purpose data-processing systems of the type schematically illustrated in Figure 4.

5
Communications and Networks

WE HAVE seen in some detail what goes to make up the hardware and software of a data processing system and have been introduced to some of the different modes of operating computers, e.g. batch operating, off-line, real time, and so on. We have considered these aspects rather in isolation, but have not considered them as systems in a closer marriage of what is possible technically and what is desirable from an organisational viewpoint. In the chapters about hardware and the history of computer development we have discussed various characteristics. In such explanations it is inevitable that an impression is given that the user organisation must conform rigidly to certain patterns and procedures that the computer system imposes. This was necessitated by the conventional wisdom which dictated that the larger the system the less the cost of the unit of work done. While obviously true, since overhead costs are better spread, it has undoubtedly led to over-investment and cumbersome systems. However, the pattern is changing. We touched on this in referring to small computers in chapter 3. The era of the enormous installation, particularly in the commercial type of application, is probably coming to a close. We still need large installations to perform long repetitive specific tasks and for 'number crunching', but such installations will be few, and they may tend to get even bigger. The user, if he is to exploit the potential of the computer, needs a more flexible interplay between his own requirements and the dictates of the machine. We should be very wary indeed of imposing rules concerning this 'interface', since such rules are inhibiting and account largely for the general air of disenchantment among users, and lack of economic justification for so many computer installations.

The most important aspect of the computer is the combination of the hardware, the software, and the needs of the application into one integrated whole: the system. It is the system aspects of computers and their use that are so neglected, so difficult, and so fascinating. It is the aspect that should most concern the user.

Without going into too much tedious detail (most of which is obvious) we have to account in a good systems design for the flow of work to and from the machine, for the organisation of the procedures to perform the work, for the maintenance of the system and for the control of costs involved in installation and running. Under these general headings we must account for a mass of detail, including data preparation and verification, program development, diagnostic routines, preventive maintenance, future expansion, operating procedures, confidentiality, and so on. All these factors must be welded together into a system pattern that will itself be thoroughly integrated into the organisation that proposes to use a computer. How far this integration goes will depend on what is expected from the system. It is for this reason that we have pleaded throughout this book for a better understanding of the principles of computer usage by all potential users. It is impossible to establish a thoroughly integrated system without deep examination of the objectives of the organisation itself. This is especially true when we talk of 'information' or, 'total systems'.

We always start from the point at which the manually operated system has brought us. Patient record handling is a typical example. The manual system has allowed the inclusion of copious hand-written notes and these notes form the most important part of the record. Some basic principles concerning patient records are discussed in the next chapter. Some years ago it was confidently thought that patient records should be forced into a pattern which would allow the bulk to be stored on a disc and thereafter be capable of being accessed randomly by anyone desiring to do so; great anxieties then arose about confidentiality. Who was going to be allowed access to the record? Was there a way of restricting this access to a few nominated individuals?

The difficulties of organising the 'inputting' of these records (their accuracy, the errors of transposition and so on) and the enormous cost involved in creating and maintaining large data banks have at least caused us to think more seriously about the different levels of information that clinicians, or nurses, or administrators need in order to perform their function in relation to the patient. This strikes at the basis of the clinical management of the patient and, once again, reinforces our oft-repeated plea. At present the Department of Health and the Scottish Home and Health Department are conducting a number of experiments in an attempt to clarify this extremely complex subject.

As we have already indicated, computer systems are becoming less costly all the time, and this applies particularly to the electronic elements—the processor, the store and the various control devices. The electro-mechanical devices such as line printers follow this pattern only very slowly. Thus, we can more readily include ample store or even extra processors in the system, if required.

At the same time, the Post Office are continually providing faster lines between points anywhere in the U.K. High-speed line connections can be made between virtually anywhere in the United Kingdom. It is true that the hire charges on these lines are high but good systems design can to some extent minimise these. The combination of these two factors: cheaper electronics and better line facilities, begin to make practical all sorts of control and management information systems that heretofore have been impractical or too costly. Moreover, such systems will allow data to be processed where they are better processed, not where the central processor happens to be. We are released from over-centralised rigid systems. This is important as it conforms to the organisational and human need to provide some autonomy at the local or regional level, yet provides a means of supervising the whole system.

We have already referred to small computers, terminals and networks. The development that is likely to have the greatest impact on Health Service computer needs is the growth in the use of terminals.

A terminal can be merely a teleprinter, but in the sense we use it here we include an input device (a teleprinter) and an output device such as a line printer. Most manufacturers offer a means of connecting these devices to a Post Office communications line. The combinations of input and output devices and a 'black box' line connector is called a 'hardwired' terminal. This provides a means of entering jobs into the system from a site remote from the central processor and is known as a remote job entry terminal. Although a terminal offers access to the processor, for many users, more conveniently than sending packs of cards by hand to the mainframe, it does result in a great increase in the 'housekeeping' load on the mainframe or central processor.

Now that processors and store are so much less costly we can employ these in the terminal itself; we can, therefore, have a 'programmable' terminal. This 'intelligent' terminal can be programmed to do a lot of the processing that would normally be done at the mainframe in the case of hardwired terminals. So the mainframe can support more intelligent terminals than hardwired terminals. More importantly, we can allocate the work to be done to the machine best suited to do the work. Most jobs presented to a processor are trivial, and many can be done by the local processor at the intelligent terminal without recourse to the mainframe. The bigger jobs can be shunted from the terminal to the mainframe, the data having been partly processed and reduced in bulk to save line hire charges.

The combinations of many small computers linked to a few large computers in well-integrated systems is the sort of way in which computers are likely to provide some solutions to the problems of information processing in the health care field generally.

The new organisation of the Health Services is largely aimed at integration of general practice, local authority health and welfare services, and the hospital service. It is not difficult to imagine how networks of small and large computers could be employed. We propose to avoid detailed descriptions of such systems since we are concerned chiefly to point out principles and characteristics. In Scotland, the Home and Health Department are already developing a network system that employs these techniques at the Medical School in Aberdeen. A regional computer network is also being developed in the Oxford region. Such networks will provide a means of controlling more effectively what goes on in the provision of health care, since the managers of the system, doctors, nurses, and administrators are more likely to be better informed about the way resources are being used.

6
Medical Records Procedures

MANAGEMENT: THE PRIME PURPOSE OF RECORD-KEEPING

MANY MILLION pieces of paper are added to medical records yearly; their compilation and servicing by doctors, nurses, records clerks and others, absorbs considerable effort. Yet, other than as an aide-memoir, and a not very efficient or infallible one at that, and as some sort of reference in the occasional medico-legal situation, they are for most practical purposes inadequate. The advent of the computer provides both the pretext and the opportunity for re-appraising the whole business, and for introducing more rational and useful procedures. Rational and useful for what? the reader may ask. It is not easy to answer this, but it involves assessing the role of medical records in patient management, ward management, hospital management, health management and medical research. What information do we need, why do we need it, how frequently do we need it, how accurately do we need it, in what form do we need it, and exactly what do we want to do with it? 'To keep it in case . . .', is surely not enough to justify the cost and effort. No, *management* is the key word, and automation, which we have defined as built-in management for enabling a system to achieve its objectives measurably and effectively, is the key to putting it on a more rational and useful basis.

A TYPICAL EXAMPLE OF COMPUTER-ASSISTED RECORD-KEEPING

The following relatively straightforward example will introduce the reader to what this means in practice. Although it relates to the somewhat specialised context of maintaining the immunity of a community at a high level (the primary objective) and as

56 *Medical Automation*

economically as possible (the secondary objective), the methods involved have the merit of being generally applicable to a wide variety of medical records procedures. What follows is an outline description (a detailed description would be out of place in this introductory text) of a system pioneered by Dr T. M. Galloway (Chief Medical Officer of Health for West Sussex) and his colleagues, some years ago in West Sussex County Council. On the birth of each child in the area, a schedule of vaccination and immunisation is agreed by the parents by signing a suitably designed pro-forma which sets out what has been agreed. In addition the form contains details of the child's address, date of birth, and the clinic or general practitioner's surgery where the parents wish the child to be dealt with. These forms, numbering many tens of thousands are converted into punched card form. A blank reel of magnetic tape is inserted into one of the computer's magnetic tape units; the punched cards are inserted into the computer's card reader; and then under the control of a suitable program the records in punched-card form are transferred to magnetic tape. These magnetic tapes, each of which can store around ten thousand such records, constitute a modern filing system. A hundred thousand records thus filed occupy little more than a cubic foot of space, and when not being used may be locked away safely in a cupboard. In fact, to guard against risk a duplicate set may be easily reproduced and kept elsewhere, a step which one could hardly contemplate with a paper records system. Moreover, there is no chance that the records will get out of order, and there is the inestimable advantage, as we shall see, that the records can be speedily 'processed' or analysed for any purpose.

In fact in this particular case, these magnetic tapes containing all the records (the 'data') are fortnightly fitted to the magnetic tape units of a computer, and a vaccination and immunisation 'appointments program' is inserted* into the central processor. The current date is also inserted into the computer via a punched card (or remote teleprinter). This is done in a matter of minutes, the start-button is pressed, and the appointments procedure is carried out entirely automatically and incredibly quickly. What the computer does, in effect, is to subtract the current date from the date on which each child had its last particular dose, which

*This, too, is kept on magnetic tape.

results in a time interval being calculated. If the interval of time is great enough the computer prints out an appointment card (pre-paid postage) with the appropriate address so that it can be posted directly. In fixing the appointment, the computer procedure will have 'looked up' the appointments record for the relevant practitioner or clinic (each of whom by arrangement allocates regular fixed periods), and chosen a convenient appointments slot. The second print-out the computer provides is an appointments list for each clinic, usually with all the 'polios' grouped together, the 'diphtherias' grouped together, and so on. A third print-out provided by the computer is a 'kits list' which sets out the materials requirements of each clinic, so that this can be delivered in good time. All this is carried out reliably in a few hours without any human effort.

In due course the appointments are (or are not) kept. The practitioner will complete the attendance information and return the attendance sheet to the computer centre. There, this new data is punched out and inserted into the computer together with an 'updating program'; the 'master file' tapes are at the same time placed in the magnetic tape units. When the start-button is pressed, each record on the magnetic tape files is appropriately updated, but, in addition, the item-by-item fees are calculated for each doctor and cheques printed for remittance, and, also, any accounts and statistical returns are assembled for the Executive Council's purposes—once again, at incredible speed and without human effort. In cases where appointments are not kept, the child's record is not updated, and at the next fortnightly 'run' an even greater interval of time will have elapsed since the child was last treated and so, automatically, another appointment is arranged. For continual non-attendance this procedure could it seems, go on being made forever. However, the computer procedure is arranged to score each appointment and after three such scores, the computer prints out a list of 'follow-ups' for the medical officer so that he can arrange for a health visitor to ascertain the reason for non-attendance. Apart from all the effort saved, the efficacy of this method of working has upgraded the population immunity from levels of around 75 per cent to more than 90 per cent, and the system has now been extended to include cervical cancer screening. Operating the system requires little skill, and is well within the scope of many clerks who at present carry out these procedures laboriously and relatively expensively by manual methods. Such skills and effort as there is, resides in the design of the computer programs. Starting from scratch, preparing the pro-formas and writing and testing the programs makes slow and tedious progress but the reward for success is both satisfying and of lasting utility.

Many other extensions are possible, but discussion of these is left for later chapters. What should be reasonably clear at this point, is how a file of records can be kept on magnetic tape and can be scanned or analysed by means of a general-purpose data-processing system of the kind illustrated in Figure 4. Without introducing any further complexity into our thinking, it is useful to consider some useful implications of having data in a form (magnetic tape) that renders it amenable to speedy analysis.

MAGNETIC TAPE FILES AND THEIR MANY POSSIBLE APPLICATIONS

The maintenance of registers of cancer, psychiatric, prenatal, orthopaedic and other patients in magnetic tape form facilitates statistical analysis and searches. Medical surveys also come into this category. How often is the scale on which data is collected in this way inhibited by the size of the time-consuming chore of the 'handraulic' analysis that must follow, and how often does the time taken to analyse such data outrun the enthusiasm and even the tenure of the teams that started the survey? Surveys are becoming a common adjunct to medical research, as it reaches back into the social and environmental factors affecting disease, and doubtless much more will be gained from them as the mechanics of analysing the data are made easier. In particular, prospective investigations can be made so quickly that less use will have to be made of retrospective analyses of existing records which only fortuitously contain data adequate for particular purposes. For example, a research worker interested in the hypothesis, say, that a certain blood group is associated with a certain type of leukaemia might request that in the geographical area of interest, blood groups be reported for every case of the particular leukaemia in question, together with any other factors needed to validate the hypothesis; this reporting need only continue until sufficient cases have been acquired. The odds are, of course, that this would eventually lead to supplementary data being required to support extensions or modifications of the original hypothesis. A similar procedure could be used to gather experimental data for a number of research workers at the same time. All this has the merit of only collecting what data is required for the purpose(s) in hand, and is so much more efficient than collecting everything on everybody 'just in case'.

Statistical returns of all sorts could be more efficiently dealt with by similar methods, and would have the benefit of being available sooner as well as so much more cheaply. With computers, however, one might well ask why wholesale statistics are needed at all. After all, nobody reads them all, if they read them at all. At the very least a computer may be used to sift statistics at regular intervals and only print out significant departures from levels previously established, thereby dispensing only what is different and therefore of interest. Increases in cross-infection, in congenital abnormalities, in levels of morbidity, in durations of stay in hospital in particular disease categories, in the incidence of particular complications, and so on, can thus be *automatically* brought to the attention of doctors and administrators a good deal sooner than might otherwise, if at all, be the case. This knowledge of current happenings, as well as of trends, both in sufficient detail to validate comparisons, will obviously assist in the management of medical care. In many cases, however, it might be better still not to produce any regular statistics (except as just described where these are wanted for monitoring a situation), and just keep the original data on magnetic tape. Specific statistics could then be readily generated to meet a specific enquiry. It is hoped that computers have removed the need for many statistical tables, which often were only generated to provide answers to questions that might arise. Too often, of course, they are unable to provide answers because the original data is either incomplete or missing.

Magnetic tape files are not only advantageous where large numbers or records are involved; they can also be used where a large quantity of data is kept on fewer patients. A cardiologist may wish to investigate the effects of anti-coagulant therapy on his coronary patients over a number of years; a surgeon to analyse the postoperative morbidity of his atrial septal defect manoeuvres; a psychiatrist might be interested in determining the diagnostic profiles of his schizophrenics, and a paediatrician might be similarly interested in his dyslexics; or a urologist may have an interest in the histological classification of testicular tumours. By keeping a reel of magnetic tape in their desk drawers, each may, by using only minutes of computer time, have their secretary or assistant update new patient data onto the file, and analyse or tabulate anything of interest. As each new hypothesis occurs it can be tested, or additional data collected for the purpose. Many hypotheses, that might otherwise remain conjectural because of the effort, can thus be examined. Files of this type can also be used to aggregate data from a number of sources in order to overcome the limitation of one man's or one department's experience. Consider an example in obstetrics. With an incidence of congenital abnormalities of about two per cent, an obstetrician delivering as many as 400 babies a year will expect to meet half-a dozen or so such cases. Suppose he met four last year and meets six this year; is this significant? Obviously not: a few is what he expects and a few is what has occurred. The fact that underlying this variation is a small but significant increase in abnormalities, due say to thalidomide, will not be revealed by this amount of experience. The argument would apply much more strongly to an obstetrician delivering only a hundred or so babies a year, and it applies not only to obstetricians and congenital abnormalities, but to any doctor with respect to the incidence of any factor of small incidence in any kind of patient.

The simple fact is that the experience of one man, however busy and able, is no longer sufficient to detect significant changes in events of low incidence which may be due to any one of a large number of factors. Patient management is cerebrally limited. Computers can help by aggregating experience. In obstetrics, for example, if a carbon copy of only a quarter of the birth records in the United Kingdom were sent to a computer centre, about 20,000 such records would be received each month, an amount that is, that would not come within the experience of an obstetrician within a life-time. From this amount of data, a computer could detect small but significant increases in abnormalities correspondingly sooner than an unaided doctor. Taking thalidomide as an example, the computer could quickly and automatically print the full details of the abnormality records so that investigations into causes and common factors could start well before any individual obstetrician was aware that there was anything significant to investigate.

Similar methods may be applied to the monitoring of new drugs. Everyone today is conscious of the fact that when all the laboratory tests, animal experiments, and clinical trials have been performed, there still exists an unknown element of risk. This serves to underline the limitation of drug protection procedures as they stand: they can only test for what the experts know they don't know; they cannot test for what the experts don't know they don't know—the real risk with anything new. Even today, with stricter rules, as a direct result of the thalidomide tragedy, expert opinion has declared itself very doubtful whether the teratogenic effects of thalidomide would have been revealed had all the new rules been in force at the time. A useful extension to existing procedures would be to make it mandatory to report on a new drug during the early stages of its introduction, together with any deleterious consequences that are subsequently found, so that this data could be systematically aggregated and analysed by computer methods. A limited area might be chosen for the first-stage introduction of a new drug. This additional surveillance would obviously alert attention at an early stage to the more harmful effects of new drugs, but it is probably the only way of correlating the less conspicuous effects, which may take some years to manifest themselves in full, with the consequent danger of the originating cause being missed entirely.

These few examples underline once again the fundamental role of information in all decision processes. A detective of high intelligence looking into a lighted window and observing only shadows will need to take shrewd account of every shred of information to glean only a vague idea of what is happening, whereas a person of no exceptional intelligence or ability able to open the curtains, will know with certainty what is going on. So it is with the doctor as compared with the computer. The latter has no powers of perception or intelligence, but when it is programmed to analyse data it can do so on a different scale and can arrive at conclusions superior in certain situations to those of human intelligence shrewdly assessing less complete information.

It will, of course, be argued how far it is practicable to collect all data on all patients simply to guard against rare occurrences. This is certainly not what is being proposed. There is no case whatever for collecting everything and storing it expensively in electronic form 'just in case', which is about as enlightened as employing a million monkeys on a million typewriters in the hope one day, of producing a sonnet. The *objectives* of the exercise should be explicit from the start: they may be to screen the introduction of new drugs, or to screen particular categories of mortality or morbidity; they may be to compare different practices on similar patients, or to maintain acceptable standards of practice; they may be to test specific hypotheses or, as in the case of vaccination and immunisation, to implement specific procedures. In all these cases *the data required for the purpose* can and must be defined, as can the data-procedures involved. The expensive ritual of storing all data in a computer, 'because it is there', and of tabulating it because it can now be tabulated, should be firmly resisted. Busy-ness and effectiveness are not always highly correlated, and this applies every bit as much to computer activity as it does to human activity.

Administrators, as we recognise, concerned with the proper and efficient use of resources, especially when overseeing vast public expenditure, must have some means of control over the money spent: the bald statistic of 'average patient stay' in our hospitals is a case in point. It is less than effective because everyone can and does argue that 'our patients are not typical'; it is a crude yardstick because 'handraulic' methods are simply too slow and cumbersome to enable more valid comparisons to be made. The 'average patient stay' is one of the main features of a regular and systematic audit of hospital activity introduced into the United Kingdom some years ago, known as Hospital Activity Analysis (H.A.A.). Essentially, it means taking into explicit account many more factors than before, such as age, sex, social class and diagnosis of patients, their source of referral, the number and type of laboratory tests made on them, details of surgery and drug therapy, clinicians in charge of the case, and so on. As it becomes fully computerised, it will enable the best practices to be identified and encouraged, and will enable approved standards of practice to be effectively monitored; it will provide a sufficiently detailed and up-to-date pattern of hospital activity to enable both the management to manage (i.e. respond to what is actually going on, particularly in relation to need and performance), and help planners to identify the medical requirements of a particular area. Some, of course, will say that such a scheme could easily degenerate into a degree of bureaucratic eavesdropping tantamount to the enthronement of 'Big Brother', and the possibility has to be admitted. Indeed it can be avoided only if medical personnel actively participate in the formulation of objectives, and understand the means by which they can be achieved; if they participate in the choice of data to be collected and the form and rate at which it needs to be collected and utilised. The medical profession will soon be unable to prevent a high degree of public and professional scrutiny, a practice long since common in other professions. Personal and subjective standards are never a substitute for measurable performance and will inevitably and inexorably be displaced by more objective assessments which computer methods make possible. The doctor-patient relationship is important for a number of good reasons, but the days in which it will remain sacred are over (Balimforth, 1972).

Even in general practice, where computers were introduced almost incidentally to assist with the process of regularly analysing prescriptions (Wade, 1968), it was found that the procedures, 'reveal useful insight about disease, patients and doctors'. This is complementary to the knowledge gained from an in-depth morbidity survey compiled from 35 general practitioners in the Exeter area (Ashford and Pearson, 1968) which suggests that a routine extended analysis of general practice, local authority, and hospital outpatient and admission activities would improve the management of community health services.

Thus, the computer is setting a trend towards a wider scrutiny of all aspects of medical practice, from data reporting systems (computerised data collection it will be recalled is only the first part of the automated management data-cycle) to more comprehensive systems of assessment and control; that is, towards computerised management information systems.

ACCURACY

All this, of course, necessitates collecting accurate data. Accuracy is solely a function of checking. The more checking the greater the accuracy, but there is no such thing as 100 per cent accuracy any more than in engineering there is such a thing as 100 per cent precision. If engineering tolerances are to be maintained within a tenth of an inch, or a hundredth of an inch, then procedures must be arranged accordingly. So it is with accuracy; it is commensurate with effort, and because effort necessitates expenditure, it is wise only to call for that degree of accuracy that will ensure the validity of whatever results are required. In other words, the accuracy of data cannot be divorced from the uses to which the data have to be put, and Rolls-Royce precision should be confined to those situations that require it.

When that is understood the role of computers is clear: it is to supply the effort. And since computers enable data to be checked automatically in ways that would otherwise be impracticable it can be asserted categorically that *the introduction of computers into medicine will do far more to improve the accuracy of medical data than any other single thing.* Errors of transcription need not be dwelt on, since there are a variety of technical procedures for reducing them to negligible proportions for most practical purposes. Errors of substance in clinical data can to a large extent be uncovered by what are commonly termed 'automatic validity checks'; these are designed in conjunction with the clinician so that any implausible, improbable, or unusual items of data are automatically referred back by the computer for confirmation or correction. For example, in obstetrics the computer can be made to refer back any patient's record in which the maternal age is outside certain limits, or in which there has been a neonatal death without a cause being stated, or in which the mother's hospital stay has exceeded the infant's without any maternal complication being reported, and so on. These clinical criteria can obviously be made as stringent as required, and it hardly needs to be said that if a doctor knows that his data are to be submitted to extensive plausibility checks of this type, then at least his records will be plausible. It is of interest in this context to report one instance in the United States where this type of checking was employed. It was found at a computing centre receiving over 300,000 prenatal records (each of some 90 items) a year from 150 hospitals, that the average rate of referral of records to hospitals which had participated in the scheme for a year or more, was less than 2 per cent, whereas it was upwards of 30 per cent for some of the new hospitals joining the scheme. This underlines a fact already stated, namely that accuracy is primarily a function of whatever degree of checking is employed; it also underlines the obvious fact that current medical records, largely unchecked, contain a lot of inaccurate data. Perhaps it is not too cynical to add that this does not matter since not much use is made of it once it gets into a typical medical records library—certainly this is true in terms of the many possible uses already referred to. In scanning and searching medical records a computer can filter off data of suitable accuracy for any specific purpose and can examine only that proportion of records satisfying specific criteria, and take only these into account in making its analyses. This should allay the fears of those who feel that there is a risk of good quality data being diluted by that of indifferent quality. This simply is not so. Even consistent mis-labelling of, say, morbidity categories can be detected by correlating morbidity levels with the persons originating the record data. This may be found to be the only factor corresponding to significantly different levels, and if so, the source of error may be identified. Hence, although at the present time medical data are not as accurately recorded as they need to be for their optimum use and although doctors differ in their classifications, this need not be a barrier to using computers successfully. In fact, computerised checking procedures can provide a measure, for the very first time, of the extent and degree to which these anomalies and shortcomings exist; a prerequisite for solving them.

CODING

When considering computerised medical records it must be recognised that a typical set of medical notes contains a very heterogeneous collection of data. By using the techniques previously described there is, in principle, no problem in storing all the information contained in a medical record in a computer, but storage by itself has little virtue (apart from compactness) compared with paper files. The main advantages we want to achieve by using computers is the ability to retrieve data selectively and speedily for particular purposes, and if this is to be done by programmed procedures, the data have to be stored in a form allowing selective retrieval and analysis. An important distinction in this context is between that data that are potentially codifiable and that which are not.

Codifiable data are 'enumerable'. For example, a patient's blood-pressure may be any of a large number of values, but the range of all such values is finite and can be enumerated. Equally, a patient may belong to any one of many disease categories, treatment categories or operation categories, but again the range can be enumerated; that is, a numerical code can be assigned to each category. On the other hand, the possible number of doctor's notes, or electrocardiograph traces is infinite. Few, if any, doctors would accept a choice from a pre-set list of enumerated sentences in place of a free-style comment; few doctors would assign a category number to a radiograph in place of seeing it; some might maintain that electroencephalographs and electro-cardiographs may be classified but not every doctor would accept another's classification. Only if agreement of this sort becomes possible for some proportion of electrocardiographs, radiographs, and so on, will they become enumerable and, hence, codifiable; meantime, it is best to recognise the fundamental distinction between codifiable and non-codifiable categories.

Broadly speaking, the art and individuality of clinical medicine is embodied in non-codifiable data, the more scientific and universally verifiable part of medicine being embodied in codifiable data. The latter is already a substantial and fast-growing part and it represents knowledge that is easily communicated and readily analysable; computers will greatly facilitate this process. Non-codifiable data will, of course, remain, but in modern medicine the trend is to move beyond highly individual personal assessments. One might even question at the present time whether all non-codifiable data are genuinely so: not all doctor's notes are that unique.

Take X-ray reports: obviously there is no limit to the possible types of X-ray report that could conceivably occur; they are infinite. But in practice an appreciable proportion of them are similar to one another. It might be that 70 per cent of all X-ray reports could be assigned to say, 120 different categories*; the remaining 30 per cent could then all be assigned to category 121. In this way one could deal with X-ray reports as codifiable (enumerable) data with all the advantages this confers for routine and research (analytical) purposes. Such reports, like all codifiable data, can be stored efficiently in computer files, and when any of the categories up to and including category 120 occurred, the clinician would know exactly what was meant, but when category 121 occurred then he would have to call for the full report in its original form. Symptoms and signs can be treated

*These figures are purely illustrative though doubtless they could be ascertained from an operational research investigation.

in a similar way by assigning those occurring most often to specific categories and pushing all others into a miscellaneous category. This would enable medical data to be analysed far more than at present.

In effect, this is questioning the alleged uniqueness of much medical data. Certainly all patients are different, even unique, but to the extent that they are unique medicine can do nothing about them. Only when a clinician can recognise similarities in histories, symptoms and signs and relating these to previous cases can assign diagnostic labels, and by hoping that the same treatment will have broadly the same effect, can he manage to help patients at all. Patients are all different, but only to the extent that there is a high element of reproducibility (implying non-uniqueness and therefore partial classifiability) is medical care possible. Progress in medical care requires a progressive increase in codifiable data at the expense of non-codifiable data, and this allows an increased use of advanced technology in the evaluation and management of the health services.

Non-codifiable data then, can only be *stored* in a computer and retrieved as required in the form in which they were inserted; it cannot be analysed; moreover, they are relatively expensive to store. Codifiable data, on the other hand, are suitable for analysis for different purposes, and are inexpensive to store. Obviously the next question is: who is going to do the irksome business of coding? In essence there are two extremes: either all the coding is undertaken manually before the data is inserted into the computer, or as much as possible is done automatically by the computer. The former has the advantage that the user satisfies himself as to the codification, and, also, that computer procedures need be designed to deal only with coded data—which allows considerable simplification; the disadvantage is the unpleasantness of coding and the fact that it retains a personal element and is thus not necessarily error-free—to err is human. The other extreme has the advantage that a major chore is eliminated, but it complicates the design of the computer procedure to include coding procedures that will operate under a wide range of linguistic variations. Most practical modern computer procedures have adopted a position between these two extremes, with the tendency of moving towards computer codification. Undoubtedly this will continue, for it makes sense to use the computer as much as possible. The difficulty *at the moment* arises principally from the nature of medical language. As Anderson (1968) has remarked—

'Most members of the medical profession have really two working medical vocabularies: one relating to general medical knowledge, skills and judgements—largely acquired at medical school—and the other a comprehensive and detailed system dealing in much more depth with the special aspects of the branch of medicine in which the doctor is practising. Thus it can be seen that few doctors cover the whole vocabulary range; most have both a very specialised and a general vocabulary.

'. . . The specialised vocabulary of the doctor continues to increase and grow, not only in its technological aspects, but also from the aspect of the type of care and management that the doctor is giving his patients. The doctor who investigates his patients in hospital requires a different vocabulary from his friend in general practice outside in the community. Problems of investigation and management have different requirements in these two areas of medical care and must be described and recorded in different ways. Practical necessity often decides the breadth and depth of any individual's medical vocabulary.

'. . . the tendency for the doctor half a century ago was still to develop a personal vocabulary with much variation, the interpretation of which, as far as management and care of patients were concerned, mattered little.

'With the rapid growth of public health and community and environmental medicine, the doctor has been forced to classify, so that preventive medicine could be translated into reality and *appropriate action be taken on the results of data obtained* (the author's italics). Thus, from the preventive and social aspects of medicine, epidemiology arose, requiring that terms be defined and data collected systematically. Community care has emphasised the need to standardise and expand the medical vocabulary in directions outside the immediate disease situation.'

Computers will reinforce this trend, and the initial attempts to computerise clinical data is focusing attention on codifiability and classifiability. One attempt is SWITCH (*S*ystem at the *W*estern *I*nfirmary, for the *T*otal *C*omputerisation of case-*H*istories). This system identifies four distinct types of data, and four 'input' computer procedures have been designed and programmed to cope with these.

The first type is that which naturally originates in numerical form, such as age, weight, height, laboratory measurements, and so on; such data presents little difficulty. The second type is that which is not intrinsically numerical, but which can be coded at the time of collection, such as commonly occurring symptoms. Because symptoms have varying levels of manifestation, their presence or absence is graded from 0 (absent) to 3 (severe); and a further qualification to the meaning is introduced by means of 'item modifiers'. For example, '75 3' opposite 'heartburn' means that heartburn recorded as severe is estimated to be only 75 per cent reliable. This weighting factor stored alongside the item in the computer can be used to modify any subsequent analysis, and can also be used verbally to qualify the symptom when the record is printed out for any reason. Obviously, such a system of coding enables the clinician to record accurately what he has observed, in contrast with what a cruder 'yes/no' scheme would permit, and there is little inconvenience in undertaking this type of coding at the time of collection. In fact, once practised, it could both shorten and refine record-taking. The third type of clinical data that is separately treated, is intended to cope with data that are intrinsically codifiable, but which would take too long to code at the time of collection. In this case the computer stores a numbered list or 'dictionary' of phrases, which might include for example, 'repair of inguinal hernia', and when this phrase is entered into the computer from the record, the computer scans the dictionary and automatically encodes the phrase. The scanning and coding procedure is rather elaborate so that each variant in the phrase is assigned a number, thus preserving any subtle differences of meaning that might arise from a particular juxtaposition of the variants in the phrase. In those cases where a phrase which does not appear in the dictionary at the time is used by a clinician, a temporary code number is assigned, and simultaneously a computer print-out indicates the fact. A decision can then be made as to whether or not to incorporate the new phrase in the dictionary. Thus, new phrases can be assimilated and the dictionary can develop continually. However, the choice of new phrases to be admitted is subject to human decision, and this is one point at which computerised dictionaries can influence the terms employed and so can impose some selectivity and discipline on the language permitted. In fact, a side-effect of SWITCH is that it will enable the frequency of use of medical terms to be ascertained, and this will have obvious value in further attempts to standardise medical terminology. The SWITCH dictionary at present (which is initially designed to cope with in-patients and out-patients suffering from peptic ulcers attending the professorial surgical unit of the Western Infirmary, Glasgow) is classified into categories for treatment, operations, diagnoses and physical signs, and has nearly 750 main phrases with over 2,000 individual variants.* The fourth category of information handled by the SWITCH system is that which is infinite and therefore intrinsically uncodifiable, namely, free comment. This is simply written out on the medical record and stored in alphabetical form in the computer; it cannot be analysed but it can be retrieved as required. In summary, therefore, medical data is classified as—

(a) numerical, which needs no coding
(b) codifiable, coded manually at the time of collection
(c) codifiable, automatically coded by the computer, and
(d) uncodifiable free comment, stored and retrieved without alteration.

It was mentioned earlier in this chapter that automatic coding complicates the design and programming of computer procedures, and it is of interest, therefore, to note that the *Lancet* paper on SWITCH records the fact that, 'Since the input programs have taken three years to write it is essential that new documents can be introduced without program alteration'. Thus, we identify a further pressure from computer application to standardise; we can elect what form of standardisation it is to be at the outset, but once a sizeable amount of programming effort has been invested in this chosen form, only the strongest of arguments are likely to influence its modification. The moral is clear: great care should be taken at the outset to ensure that the format chosen for medical records procedures is suitable.

The SWITCH system designers propose an attractive solution

*This may be compared with Anderson's comment in the paper already cited, that, 'The standard medical vocabulary being developed at King's College, Hospital, London, has about 30,000 terms at present and probably needs to be expanded still more to become adequate in all medical specialties. Certainly this means that the average general working medical vocabulary we expect the medical student and doctor to know by the time he qualifies is about 15,000–20,000 terms.'

to solving the generality of uses to which medical records may be put, by basing their approach on modularity. A programming module is designed for each general section of data, thus enabling programmes to be built up to handle 'any document provided it is built up from general sections'. There are 24 such sections at the present time, and doubtless their suitability to cope with the wide variety of medical situations will be tested in the next few years. Significantly, in view of the earlier comments in this chapter, they do go on to remark that—

> 'While it is expected that specialised clinics, like the peptic ulcer clinic, will have most of its clinical information in a coded form, less specialised clinics, such as a general medical clinic, will at first have only a small proportion of the history in a strictly defined form while the rest will be handled as free comment. However, it is likely that the amount of information in descriptive English will gradually decrease as the advantages of having precisely defined information stored in computers becomes obvious.'

PATIENT IDENTIFICATION

One of the characteristic features of computers is that they sharpen focus on problems that hitherto have tended to drift along in their own sweet way. Already we have been made to think about what data are really needed, why they are needed, what purpose statistics serve, and we have needed to think more carefully about accuracy and coding. Another problem that has occasioned a considerable amount of thought on the part of those feeling their way in medical computer application is that of patient identification.

The crux of the problem is now familiar, namely that computers can only process *structured* data; they have no ability to deal with *meaning*. Yet patient identification data is as unstructured as any. Names can vary (Jim, Jimmy, James), first and second names can become transposed and abbreviated, surnames can change (particularly on marriage), addresses can vary in style (47 London Road, versus The Grange, 47 London Road), they get abbreviated, transposed with a variety of punctuation, and, of course, they change. To the human records clerk, these problems of meaning are usually soluble with some effort and ingenuity.

But computers, being machines, cannot hunt round meanings, they can only examine structure character by character, depending on the format.

Therefore, the problem posed is what particular structure could be adopted, and this involves multiple considerations. Is the primary objective to identify a patient within a ward, a clinic, a hospital, a general practice or the regional or national community? What is the relative efficiency of using names, dates of birth, sex, and so on, none of which is individually unique? How acceptable are truncated names that fit into a fixed format? How confusing this would be to the least skilled workers, such as porters, junior nurses, theatre attendants and ambulance drivers? How readily would a chosen structure lend itself to automatic data-processing, and so on? A great deal of thought has been given to these problems over the past decade, starting with pioneer work on records-linkage by Newcombe and others in Canada and by Acheson in this country. Newcombe showed that the most accurate items to use in patient identification are surname at birth, and mother's maiden name, but for a number of reasons these are not the most practical items to use in general patient identification. Because labels must be used at various times by general practitioners, telephonists, porters and ambulance drivers, as well as by relatives and friends accompanying patients, Dale and Roberts in a detailed study (Dale and Roberts, 1968) gave the opinion that name and address are essential. Moreover, they agreed with colleagues in the Birmingham Teaching Hospitals that

> 'all personal and record identification items should be collected on registration of in-patients at the hospital; and that the computer input should be created as a by-product of normal recording procedures. In view of this the labels for identification within the special hospital population had to be a sub-set of those for identification within the wider population'.

On names in particular, Dale and Roberts found that a survey of 1,745 surnames of patients registered in their hospital indicated that thirteen letters would cover all but one in 10,000 names, and no forename of more than eleven characters was found in a dictionary of British Forenames. They felt, therefore, that a fixed format for names should be adopted, comprising thirteen letters for surname, eleven for forename and three for the second name. Details of the other items they chose for patient identification in their projects are set out in detail in the reference given above. Others, doubtless, will argue the advantages of alternative preferences for their particular purposes.

Perhaps, in time, and with the greater use of integrated record systems for multiple purposes which seems likely to come, a standardised form for patient identification will evolve. Suffice it to say that during the fluid situation that exists at the present time, decisions as to what form of patient identification to adopt, require particular care. They need to take account not only of the prime purposes to which computerised records systems will be put, but also of other uses that may subsequently arise.

We have in this chapter given a general idea of the sort of problems involved in medical record handling, and described some applications. It has often been advocated in the past that the medical record problem could be solved by putting all records on random access discs and have such a data bank accessible by visual display units throughout the hospital. At least one DHSS computer experiment is based on this general concept. Such solutions, however, are expensive and in the stringent financial climate that will always prevail in the Health Service it is extremely unlikely that money on the scale needed to put every patient record on disc will ever be available. Current expenditure on medical records in the Hospital Service is very modest and is unlikely to be increased by a factor of 10 or more in the next decade.

REFERENCES

Anderson, J. (1968) The computer: Medical vocabulary and information. *British Medical Bulletin*, **24**, 194 198.

Ashford, J. R. and Pearson, N. G. (1968) The Exeter Community Health Project, in *Computers in the Service of Medicine*. London: Oxford University Press.

Balmforth, G. V. (1972) Decision-making in clinical practice—criteria of physicians effectiveness, in *Spectrum 71*. London: Butterworth.

Dale, J. W. and Roberts, J. L. (1968) The identification of patients and their records in a hospital, in *Computers in the Service of Medicine*. London: Oxford University Press.

Wade, O. L. (1968) The computer and drug prescribing, in *Computers in the Service of Medicine*. London: Oxford University Press.

7
Computer-assisted Diagnosis

DIAGNOSIS: AN INFORMATION PROBLEM

Doctors, generally speaking are not magicians. Whatever their patients may hope or expect from them, or whatever some doctors may believe concerning their powers, they can at best do no more than medical knowledge at any given time permits, namely *to identify a patient as belonging to one or other of the known treatable categories, and to apply one or other of the known treatments for the category* (or categories) identified. This may sound simple enough, and so it was up to a few generations ago when a single person of average competence could have reasonably complete knowledge of a particular clinical situation. This fact, coupled with the unquestioning faith and lack of education of the masses who were disposed to accept God's will philosophically and medical counsel uncritically, meant that doctors were able to enjoy an authority and an autonomy which was matched only by their (relative to today) ineffectiveness.

Science and technology have changed this situation out of all recognition, starting with the introduction of anaesthesia and microbiology about a century ago. The extent and range of medical knowledge have increased so rapidly that one doctor, however able and experienced, can know only a small part of what is medically possible. It is no longer a simple matter to categorise a patient, as there are upwards of 30,000 treatable categories which are continually being added to and modified, and no single clinician can hope to have detailed knowledge of more than a few per cent. In fact, multi-disciplinary work by medical and scientific specialists, who often work in different places, is commonly required to identify the relevant category and to treat the patient. The consequences of delays in communication, inaccuracies, ambiguities, divided responsibility, omissions (inadvertent and otherwise) and inefficiencies inherent in any attempt by cerebrally limited human organisation to bring all relevant medical skills to bear on a patient's case cannot be assessed easily. Most clinicians acknowledge that while doing their best, they can never be sure that they know everything about a certain disease. The vapour trail characteristics of human memory in which knowledge attenuates with time, the difficulties of keeping up-to-date and the limited retentive capacity of the brain, all mitigate against it. In practice, it is no longer medical knowledge limiting what is medically possible, but the means of bringing the relevant parts of it to bear on a particular clinical situation. The *potential* effectiveness of medicine in fact is far greater than it was, but the *information* and *communication* problems associated with realising this potential are insuperable by the unaided cerebral cortex. The problem has been growing for some years now and with the continued growth of medical and scientific knowledge it will get more acute, unless some way can be found of assisting or extending the information processing capacity of the cerebral cortex—and for the reasons already set out this is what, in spite of difficulties, motivates the search for computer-assisted diagnostic procedures.

Of course, such a quest arouses widespread opposition. Some people oppose it on grounds of robot-medicine—a forgivable and understandable misconception; some oppose it because it will affect the traditional doctor-patient relationship—which it will, but not adversely; some oppose it on the grounds that nothing can come of it until the understanding of disease and its diagnosis are improved—almost certainly a too pessimistic appraisal for reasons to be discussed; and, finally, some oppose it in the tradition of those who have opposed innovation throughout the course of medical history, such as those who scorned Jenner's vaccination experiments, those who derided mesmerism when it was one of the few ways of alleviating pain during surgery, those who stigmatised Simpson's early attempts at anaesthesia, those who bitterly attacked Lister's antiseptic procedures, and those who trenchantly contested Pasteur's remarkable discoveries.

But prejudice should not worry us in this context as a computer imposes no particular solution to the quest for computer-assisted diagnosis. It is, as we have already learned, a machine for carrying out *whatever data-procedures, based on whatever methods,* we choose to think might be helpful, and in devising such methods we know that we do not need to be inhibited by either the amount of data involved or the amount of 'processing' (searching, comparing, weighting and possibly calculating) required of it. Nor does any method we choose have to be mathematical in character, as has been suggested: 'Analysis of this (diagnostic) process in such a way that at least a major part of it can be performed by a mathematical technique is an essential preliminary to the use of a computer (Scadding, 1967). Computers have liberated us from mathematics, which happens to be one narrow category of data-processing. Those who maintain their prejudices when the field of enquiry and possibility is so wide, are merely declining to explore the ways in which data-technology may help in making more effective use of medical knowledge. The suggestions in this chapter should, therefore, be regarded as an attempt to delineate a few possible approaches, and if it stimulates the newcomer to begin to think his own way through, it will have achieved its objective. No one can predict what the outcome of these explorations will be in ten to twenty years time; it is highly unlikely that information processing and technology will not have a profound effect on medical practice as it currently exists.

THE CONCEPT OF AN AUTOMATIC LIBRARY FACILITY

The provision of an automatic library facility would greatly benefit a clinician who could then quickly and easily bring his knowledge of differential diagnosis and treatment up to date. In general terms this might be done as follows. Suppose Dr A has certain items of information, I_1, I_2, I_3 and I_4 (which may be symptoms, signs, test-results, and so on), regarding a patient's condition and that he requires more information on the differential diagnosis than his own knowledge and experience affords. Normally, in an attempt to extend the bounds set by his own cerebral faculties, supposing he had enough time, he would consult his colleagues and the medical literature, but in addition it is now proposed that he should consult the Automatic Library Facility (ALF). This is a computer installation, perhaps with remote terminals, which could be situated in a medical centre, and in its most elementary form stores a 'disease directory' in the form of a table of disease categories (D_1 up to D_{200}, say) versus items (I_1 up to I_{100}, say). It is managed by a human operator, effectively a librarian, who may be approached directly or by telephone (or the computer system may be interrogated directly by means of a remote terminal). Asked for the very first time by Dr A which diseases are associated with I_1, I_2, I_3 and I_4, ALF will answer none, which, of course, is no great help to Dr A who can himself think of two such diseases, D_1 and D_2. ALF stores these two. When next asked a similar question by Dr B, ALF produces D_1 and D_2, one of which is news to Dr B, who notes, however, that ALF has omitted a third possibility, D_3. ALF stores D_3 in addition to D_1 and D_2, associating all three diseases with items I_1, I_2, I_3, I_4; in effect, ALF now 'knows' the associations of Drs A and B. Clearly, after one hundred doctors have enquired of ALF, the associations stored by the computer will represent the aggregate knowledge of one hundred doctors on this subject. Thereafter, ALF's suggestions will contain some very useful data because unless a doctor knows as much as *all previous enquirers*, ALF will provide new information.

In such a way, although as we shall see shortly, practical considerations require a more systematic approach, ALF could graduate from the status of an amusement (which is how most of the successful attempts to date have been regarded) to something of practical value. Indeed, the idea has already been extended so that ALF not only produces a differential diagnosis (which may be rather vague in the early stages of investigation) but also indicates what additional symptoms/signs/tests/measurements should be sought to differentiate the likely possibilities more clearly. Furthermore, since it is a straightforward matter to associate relevant treatments and prognoses with the stored disease profiles, then ALF can readily provide such information along with the differential diagnosis. From a practical point of view, in fact, this information *relating to the action to be taken* is of primary importance, since unequivocal diagnoses as such, dependent on the concept of a disease (discussed below) are not always attainable. In the role described, the ALF-procedure is discharging the function of a useful colleague. The main difference, of course, and its potential significance if it can be realised can hardly be overstated, is that ALF's knowledge has been carefully assembled and sifted from the best and most up-to-date knowledge available in each medical specialty, and is regularly reviewed to include refinements and re-definitions.

For example, if a cardiologist, say, wished to set up an Automatic Library Facility starting from scratch for his own purposes, he could start by setting down on paper the differentiating syndromes for each of a number of cardiological conditions. By a differentiating syndrome we mean all the information (symptoms, signs, age, sex, measurements, and so on) he would need to satisfy himself of the existence of a particular condition to the reasonable exclusion of all others. This table of cardiological conditions versus differentiating items (collectively the 'disease profiles') would then be stored in a computer to form a pilot cardiological ALF. Now, when a particular patient presents his symptoms, signs and so on, these can be listed and inserted into the computer (possibly via a remote-terminal) and the computer could evaluate an index of similarity or difference* between what has been observed and what is expected for each cardiological condition. It would order these indices and print out the most likely possibilities in order of probability, together with the items (symptoms, signs, tests) which would most efficiently further clarify the situation. Once additional information was obtained by the clinician, the whole procedure could be repeated, enabling ALF to make a re-assessment of the most likely possibilities in the light of the increased evidence. Repetitions would continue until sufficient confidence in the diagnosis was obtained, when the cardiologist could request information on the appropriate treatment(s) and prognosis.

Note that the computer is not making a decision; it is merely retrieving automatically all those conditions compatible with the evidence presented to it, which the clinician has elicited. To the extent that the computer 'library' has been assembled from the most comprehensive and up-to-date information available, not from one cardiologist but from many, its selection of the most likely possibilities will be based on a wider compass of knowledge than that available to any particular cardiologist. Moreover, in making its selection of all relevant diagnostic categories available, it advises on what *action* will be most valuable in guiding the cardiologist to arrive at his own (better informed) decisions.

*The nature of these indices is the essence of the problem; to date they have had a pronounced statistical bias, but until a more logical basis for clinical diagnosis exists better progress may be made by quantitative empirical indices (discussed later) which refine existing methods, rather than displace them by logical models.

We should bear in mind that what has been described is simply one method of approach out of many that one might choose to adopt. Its objective is to exploit the large data storage capacity of the computer, together with its phenomenal speed of search, to increase the relevant information available to clinicians in making their decisions. The obvious point of interest is how far this objective can be realised in practice.

The Automatic Library Facility: An Example

The authors and their colleagues at the Medical Automation Experimental Unit, University College Hospital, London, successfully demonstrated a pilot ALF as long ago as 1964. Initially, it confined itself to the limited problem of bacteriological identification, and its use in this context will serve as a useful step in explaining how it was used subsequently for computer-assisted diagnosis. Identification of bacteria is done by submitting a specimen to a number of tests the results of which give a limited number of possibilities, and then carrying out further tests sequentially for further differentiation until identification has been established to the bacteriologist's satisfaction. In the pilot ALF referred to, a table consisting of some 20 test results for each of 40 bacteria was stored in the computer (the 'directory of bacteriological profiles') and the following procedure established. A bacteriologist telephones the results of several tests performed; this data is inserted into the computer together with a 'bacteriological identification' program which, in effect, compares the particular results with those listed in each of the 40 bacteriological profiles, and evaluates an index of similarity in each case. The whole procedure takes a matter of seconds, and the computer then prints out the list of bacteria in order of the similarity index. Usually, only the first few are of any interest, and the program is designed to suppress (on request) the printing of the whole list. The computer also prints out which tests will most efficiently clarify the situation further. The following example shows the *actual* form of print-out that results from supplying it with an initial five test results.

COMPUTER-ASSISTED BACTERIOLOGICAL IDENTIFICATION

GIVEN:
INDOL	NEGATIVE
UREA	NEGATIVE
DEXTROSE	ACID
LACTOSE	NO CHANGE
MANNITOL	ACID

THEN APPLYING THESE RESULTS TO THE COMPLETE SET OF BACTERIA, THE MOST LIKELY ARE, IN ORDER OF PREFERENCE:

	Relative Likelihood (%)
SAL. TYPHI	100
SAL. GALLINARUM	100
SAL. GALLINARUM VAR DUISBERG	100
SH. FLEXNERI	52
SH. BOYD II	52
KLEBS. RHINOSCLEROMA	50

THE FOUR BEST TESTS FOR DISTINGUISHING BETWEEN THESE POSSIBILITIES ARE, IN ORDER OF PREFERENCE:

	Relative Discriminating Power
SODIUM CITRATE	1·0
XYLOSE	0·8
RHAMNOSE	0·8
DULCITOL	0·8

From this statement, as produced directly by the computer, it can be seen that there are half-a-dozen bacteria consistent with the data provided, and that the computer lists four tests that will most efficiently differentiate between them. This information is passed on to the bacteriologist who is still waiting on the telephone. The next day, when he has obtained additional test-results, the computer procedure is re-run, and produces the following print-out—

COMPUTER-ASSISTED BACTERIOLOGICAL IDENTIFICATION

GIVEN:
INDOL	NEGATIVE
UREA	NEGATIVE
SODIUM CITRATE	NEGATIVE
XYLOSE	NO CHANGE
DEXTROSE	ACID
LACTOSE	NO CHANGE
MANNITOL	ACID
RHAMNOSE	NO CHANGE
DULCITOL	NO CHANGE

THEN APPLYING THESE RESULTS TO THE COMPLETE SET OF BACTERIA, THE MOST LIKELY ARE, IN ORDER OF PREFERENCE:

	Relative Likelihood (%)
SH. FLEXNERI	100
SH. BOYD II	100
SAL. TYPHI	100
SH. DYSENTERIAE, TYPE I	20

THE FOUR BEST TESTS FOR DISTINGUISHING BETWEEN THESE POSSIBILITIES ARE, IN ORDER OF PREFERENCE—

	Relative Discriminating Power
ARABINOSE	1·0
SORBITOL	1·0
MOTILITY	0·9
MR	0·9

As before, this information is passed on to the bacteriologist, who in this example returned a further four test results on the third day. When these were inserted into the computer the results were as follows—

COMPUTER-ASSISTED BACTERIOLOGICAL IDENTIFICATION

GIVEN:

	INDOL	NEGATIVE
	MOTILITY	POSITIVE
	UREA	NEGATIVE
	SODIUM CITRATE	NEGATIVE
	MR	POSITIVE
	XYLOSE	NO CHANGE
	DEXTROSE	ACID
	LACTOSE	NO CHANGE
	MANNITOL	ACID
RHAMNOSE	RHAMNOSE	NO CHANGE
	DULCITOL	NO CHANGE
	ARABINOSE	ACID
	SORBITOL	ACID

THEN APPLYING THESE RESULTS TO THE COMPLETE SET OF BACTERIA, THE MOST LIKELY ARE IN ORDER OF PREFERENCE—

	Relative Likelihood (%)
SAL. TYPHI	100
SH. BOYD II	2
SH. FLEXNERI	1

THE BEST TESTS FOR DISTINGUISHING BETWEEN THESE POSSIBILITIES, ARE IN ORDER OF PREFERENCE—

	Relative Discriminating Power
SUCROSE	1·0
H_2S	0·9

At this stage the bacteriologist was satisfied that *Salmonella typhi* was the correct answer, and it is interesting to observe that the computer indicates that this result is fifty times more likely, on the evidence, than any other.

This is typical of many results obtained using this procedure, which consistently gave the correct answer. Moreover, the number of tests it required was generally less (as might be expected from a more quantitative approach) than the number used by the bacteriologist, thereby saving cost and time in the laboratory, as well as speeding diagnosis in some proportion of cases.

That this first attempt should have worked as well as it did should surprise no one, as it is simply a quantitative refinement of what a bacteriologist does in practice. What he does, in fact, is to compare mentally the results of tests on a particular specimen with those characteristic of all bacteria likely to be present in such a specimen. This procedure is essentially a method of qualitative analysis aided by experience and prior knowledge of the probable results. The computer merely quantifies this procedure. For example, if bacterium A is known to give a positive response to a particular test T on a proportion p of occasions, while a bacterium B is known to give a positive response to the same test on only proportion q of occasions, then on the basis of this one test it is reasonable to assign likelihoods of p and q respectively to bacteria A and B. In fact, p and q are numerical refinements of the qualitative weighting factors used by the bacteriologist. For each particular test result there will be a corresponding weighting function for every bacterium, and this determines the relative likelihood of each bacterium for each particular test (in fact 'likelihood' as used here is simply what is usually known as the 'specificity' of the test). The only problem is how to combine these likelihoods to give a compound likelihood for a number of tests. The reader may judge for himself how this is performed qualitatively: how does a bacteriologist decide between a bacterium which is 70 per cent likely on the basis of one test and 50 per cent likely on the basis of another test, compared with a bacterium that is 80 per cent and 30 per cent likely on the basis of the same two tests? Then consider how he manages to choose between some 40 bacteria each having its own specificity (likelihood) to each of a dozen tests, and one can see how 'wishy-washy' a qualitative assessment must inevitably be. Proceeding quantitatively, on the other hand, we may choose to combine the individual weighting factors *in any way that produces consistently good results*. In practice it was found that simple multiplication of the individual weighting factors worked well, and this simple algorithm (rule) will suffice until poor results dictate some change. It so happens that this procedure closely corresponds to one associated with a stricter concept of 'likelihood' as used in mathematical statistics, and from this point of view a number of criticisms of the suitability of the algorithm can be put forward, and refinements or alternative algorithms suggested. Any complication of the model that does not yield measurably better results should be resisted. Of course, eventually it is likely that every logical sophistication may be found necessary as computer-assisted procedures extend and refine their range of application; but it should be noted that a simple quantitative procedure amply refines the 'wishy-washy' nature of purely mental assessments.

This will suffice for the newcomers to whom this book is directed. (The purists will find a fuller discussion and copious references in the *British Medical Bulletin*, September 1968, entitled 'Computing in Medicine' and in Chapter 7 of *Spectrum* 1971: Report on Conference on Medical Computing: Butterworths.) A similar simple quantitative refinement is used by the computer in selecting additional tests to differentiate further between the most likely possibilities.

The whole exercise, however, takes on a new dimension when one remembers that the storage capacity of a modern computer is not limited to storing information on only 40 bacteria, as in the above example; it can just as readily store all test outcomes for every known bacterium and virus so that its reference set approximates to what is known rather than what a particular individual can recall. New data concerning pathogens could be entered into ALF by laboratories of the highest competence, whose responsibility it would be to review the entire 'data-bank' from time to time to check its accuracy. Professional personnel would keep data on pathogens up-to-date and any individual would have telephone access to the most comprehensive knowledge available, so it would be unwise to ignore the computer's 'decision'. With such a system there is less need to rely on art and hunch, which are only required when one cannot quickly and systematically scan all the relevant information. Art, hunch, and feel are cerebral makeshifts for deficiencies in memory capacity; they note a clue here and associate it with an ill-remembered event there. Experience has accumulated an untidy jumble of information, attenuated in focus by the dust of time; it is personal and subjective in character, lacking any quantitative precision. Machines can extend the capacity, extend the precision, and enhance the structuring of our collective experience, so that no longer need we rely on one leaky memory-full of experience to deploy the extensive and widening range of medical knowledge.

COMPUTER-ASSISTED DIAGNOSIS: AN EXAMPLE

In the more general case where automatic library procedures are applied not to bacteriological identification but to what we might term 'diagnostic category identification' or 'treatment category identification', the reader may wonder how it is possible to deal with vague items such as lumps, aches, and so on, which are apparently a very different kind of entity from the highly specific tests used in bacteriological identification. We know that, for example, the same lump may be described by one clinician as large, by another as small, and by another as of no importance; and in published descriptions of a particular condition a lump may be recorded as invariably present, infrequently present, or as irrelevant. Certainly 'observer error' is a very characteristic feature of medicine, and as a result it must be acknowledged that clinicians' conclusions are inevitably as disparate as their observations—computers or not. The pertinent question, therefore, is whether computers can cope with this situation at all, and if so, whether they can offer any improvement. The answers in both cases is yes.

The situation can be dealt with by using clinical statistics, which may show for example, that in a particular condition a lump has been reported as significant in 750 cases out of 1,000. This incidence ratio of 3 to 1 compares with an incidence ratio of perhaps 30 to 1 which would arise in the case of a highly specific test. We should, therefore, regard this weighting factor as a measure of the usefulness of the information contained in the highly specific test as compared with the less specific information supplied by the lump. Many more signs/symptoms/tests of low specificity (such as the lump above) will be required to underwrite a confident decision as compared with the results of a highly specific test, which in the example above will fail to be elicited in only one case out of thirty, but there is no doubt whatsoever that *they can both be taken into account on the same rational basis.*

In fact, the relative specificity of symptoms, signs and test results, and so on, alone makes diagnosis possible. All would be simple if a unique symptom, sign or test outcome characterised each disease, and none other, but, of course, it is not so. The evidence of certain items of high relative specificity will dispose the clinician to favour some possibilities rather than others, but they may not be conclusive, and items of less relative specificity may have to be weighed in order to underwrite sufficient confidence in one diagnostic conclusion rather than another. But the obvious limitations of this procedure when undertaken mentally are exactly similar to those already mentioned in the context of bacteriological identification, namely that no clinician has anything like an awareness of *all* the diseases in which a particular symptom, sign or test outcome may arise, let alone any quantitative awareness of weighting factors (relative specificities); and even if he had, how could he possibly *compound* these with any *precision*. Experience helps, but intrinsic mental shortcomings set a serious limit on how far this can be attained. Happily, it is just these limitations which the ALF-concept can overcome, since it relies essentially on storing disease-profiles in which each item is weighted with its relative specificity derived from carefully collected clinical statistics (i.e. aggregate experience). These weighting factors can then be compounded in the simple way described earlier, enabling the ALF-procedure to retrieve the most likely possibilities *and* indicate which further items will most efficiently further clarify the situation. In concept it is not ambitious; it simply compounds *numerate* relative specificitus derived from experience; it does not attempt a mathematical or statistical model of the diagnostic process; it is simply refining with numbers what mental processes only achieve qualitatively.

The following example supports this reasoning. It concerns the differential diagnosis of thyroid cancer, non-toxic goitre and Hashimoto's disease, and makes *use of exactly the same computer procedure* as that used above for bacteriological identification. The three 'disease profiles' stored in the computer were made up of some 31 items, comprising symptoms (duration of goitre, presence or absence of discomfort, pain, hoarseness, dysphagia, and so on), signs (size and consistency of thyroid gland, fixation to surrounding tissues, laryngeal palsy, and so on), test outcomes (thyroidal uptake of radio-iodine, serum protein-bound iodine measurements, and so on), and age. Each age, symptom, sign and test outcome was limited to a three-way classification, since it was felt that nothing appreciably different would be achieved by a finer classification. To provide the weighting factors, statistics were compiled from records of 53 patients with Hashimoto's disease, 51 patients with thyroid cancer, and 51 with simple goitre, in every one of whom the diagnoses had been confirmed by histological examination of thyroid tissue obtained at operation or biopsy. These three profiles, quantitatively weighted in respect of their characteristic items, made up the disease directory.

An attempt was then made to get the computer to classify a further 88 patients on the basis of their age symptoms, signs and test outcomes. A typical result is shown below—

COMPUTER-ASSISTED DIFFERENTIAL DIAGNOSIS

GIVEN: DISCOMFORT IN GOITRE   NO
        FIXATION   YES
        CERVICAL LYMPH NODES   IMPALPABLE
        PYRAMIDAL LOBE   ABSENT
        HOARSENESS   YES
        DYSPHAGIA   YES
        CHOKING OR TIGHTNESS   NO
        COUGH OR STRIDOR   YES
        MODULAR OR DIFFUSE   DIFFUSE
        DURATION (YRS)   1 to 10
        ESTIM. SIZE   0 to 100
        CONSISTENCY   FIRM
        CLINICAL STATUS   HYPOTHYROID
        AGE   30 to 60

THEN COMPARING THESE OBSERVATIONS WITH THOSE EXPECTED FOR EACH CONDITION IN TURN, THE MOST LIKELY ARE, IN ORDER OF PREFERENCE

	Relative Likelihood (%)
HASHIMOTO'S DISEASE	100
NON-TOXIC GOITRE	3
THYROID CANCER	0

THE MOST IMPORTANT ITEMS WHICH SHOULD NOW BE SOUGHT IN ORDER TO DIFFERENTIATE FURTHER BETWEEN THESE POSSIBILITIES ARE:

	Differentiating Power
THYMOL TURBIDITY	1·0
E.S.R.	0·8
GAMMA GLOBULIN	0·8
PB 131 I	0·8
RECENT INCREASE IN SIZE	0·7
PAIN IN GOITRE	0·5

Using the method of relative likelihood, which essentially involves multiplication of the relevant weighting factors as described earlier, the results obtained by Boyle and his colleagues for the 88 patients with non-toxic goitre were as follows—

	Hashimoto's disease	Simple goitre	Thyroid cancer
Clinical diagnosis correct Calculated diagnosis correct	26	21	16
Clinical diagnosis correct Calculated diagnosis wrong	2	3	0
Clinical diagnosis wrong Calculated diagnosis correct	12	0	0
Clinical diagnosis wrong Calculated diagnosis wrong	3	2	3
Number of patients	43	26	19

In effect, therefore, there was complete agreement between the clinical diagnoses and the computer-assisted diagnoses in 71 out of the 88 cases; in 5 other cases the clinician was correct, and in the remaining 12 the computer was correct, as confirmed by histological examination of thyroid tissue. All the clinicians participating in the study had at least three years' specialised experience in dealing with disorders of the thyroid.

A modification of this simple method, which has been adopted by numerous groups attempting similar studies, is to take account of what are called 'prior probabilities'. The reasoning behind this procedure is to say that if a patient is drawn at random from a population in which the prevalence of disease A is twice that of disease B, then without knowing anything at all about the patient, he is twice as likely *a priori* to have disease A; hence the likelihoods of diseases as previously worked out should be modified by the prior probabilities of the diseases in question. In their very thorough study, Boyle and his colleagues also evaluated this so-called 'Bayesian' approach (named after the Reverend T. Bayes who devised this particular statistical method in 1763) and the results they obtained were as follows—

	Hashimoto's disease	Simple goitre	Thyroid cancer
Clinical diagnosis correct Calculated diagnosis correct	26	22	13
Clinical diagnosis correct Calculated diagnosis wrong	2	2	3
Clinical diagnosis wrong Calculated diagnosis correct	12	0	0
Clinical diagnosis wrong Calculated diagnosis wrong	3	2	3
Number of patients	43	26	19

In this case the clinical and computer diagnoses agree in 69 cases; the clinician is correct in 7 of the remaining cases as compared with the computer's 12. But the computer has failed to pick up three cases of thyroid cancer which were identified by the clinician.

Boyle *et al.* comment that the slightly poorer results arising from the Bayesian approach are probably due to inaccuracies in calculation of prior probabilities of disease occurrences which may vary according to the population from which the patient is drawn. A stronger objection to this 'model' is that the commoner diseases (having a higher prior probability) are favoured in relation to the rarer diseases (having a lower prior probability) *without considering the evidence at all.* It means, in effect, that the objective clinical evidence pertaining to the rarer disease has to offset the disadvantage of its lower prior probability before it is considered equally probable. However, it is only fair to add that when one considers the details of more elaborate statistical models there is ample room for controversy in arguing the advantage of one set of assumptions over another, and the reader is best referred to the more detailed papers to form his own judgement. One weakness of the simple likelihood procedure, is that simple multiplication only produces a sensible ordering of the most likely possibilities if the items characterising the disease are reasonably independent of each other. Where this is not the case some distortion can arise unless care is taken to allow for the interdependence.

It is quite remarkable that *a first attempt* at computer-assisted differential diagnosis of non-toxic goitre should in the 88 cases to which it is applied, give better results than those of clinicians with more than three years' specialised experience. The basic facts, however, should neither alarm nor surprise since (*a*) the method simply consists of compounding relative specificities quantitatively instead of qualitatively, and (*b*) if the procedure were seen as assisting the clinician rather than as displacing him or even competing with him; that is, *if the clinician had referred to and obtained the additional information from the computer before making his diagnosis, then his final decisions would have been better* than either his alone or the computer's alone. This result confirms the suggestion that *additional* information from computer-assisted procedures can improve medical decision-making; and if it can do it in this specialised context, it can do it *a fortiori* where less-specialised clinical skill is available. This is a vivid demonstration of the more general point previously made that where computer-procedures can be devised to give a performance comparable with the most skilled and highly trained doctors it enables the less skilled and well-trained to maintain a high standard of operating practice.

TOWARDS MORE COMPREHENSIVE COMPUTER-ASSISTED DIAGNOSIS

Moving from such promising beginnings to more comprehensive

schemes of computer-assisted diagnosis has proved to be slow for a number of reasons, of which the most important is the rate at which medicine can assimilate numerate methodology. The past record of medical history in accepting innovation is not good, but the ethos of the age of change, and the inevitability of introduction of the new methods, may well move things along rather faster than some would like. Education is crucial. The task cannot be undertaken by computer scientists alone, but requires medically qualified people in every specialty to have a basic understanding of the principles involved and sufficient enthusiasm and time to take a fresh look at existing practices and co-operate with interdisciplinary teams in the development of practical schemes. Such capable all-rounders are likely to be rare and certainly up-and-coming rather than established and they will initially have to create their own opportunities within the prevailing medical career structure. Also, they will need access to expensive resources, of equipment and manpower (systems analysts and programmers), and applications for these resources will have to compete with more familiar projects, which are likely to be favoured until established thinking has assimilated more prosaic computer applications.

The feature of computer-assisted diagnostic procedures which has demonstrated its real worth has been the quantitative weighting factors derived from clinical statistics of incidence extracted from case records. Since this requires a great deal of time and skilled effort to do properly, it is not surprising that to date, computer-assisted diagnostic procedures have been confined to the differential diagnoses of a limited range of diseases. Indeed, it is difficult to see how medicine, organised as it is at the present time, with individuals in particular specialities as its focal points, can embark on collecting data to provide more comprehensive automatic library facilities. *Progress is most likely to come indirectly* from the development of computer-assisted medical records procedures, which seem harmless and so arouse less emotion. This will inevitably impose far greater discipline on the way data is collected, coded, recorded and classified; moreover, it is directing attention at what data are collected and why they are collected. We know that one of the essential objectives of patient management is the identification of the disease category, and hence it is likely that medical records will eventually contain identifying data (symptoms, signs, test results, and so on) in a structured form that lends itself more readily to computer processing. In that case *it will be possible to obtain clinical statistics of incidence without any human effort.* (Hospital Activity Analysis, is itself a first step in this direction.) Specialists will then, for the first time, be able to compare their weighting factors with each other, and will be able to observe on a continuing basis how they change with time. Once this stage of objectivity (hitherto unknown) is reached, it is only a small step to compound the weighting factors in some way to arrive at computer-assisted diagnostic decisions.

From this point of view every computer-assisted medical records project is a possible starting point towards the objective of computer-assisted diagnosis. Some will find the going easier than others by virtue of their specialised path, and others will doubtless meet considerable obstacles on the way; some may feel that it will be a far happier experience to travel than to arrive. But the prime motivation should not be forgotten: the benefit to the patient if all relevant information can be more readily and efficiently utilised.

A great deal of discussion about the diagnostic process and the concept of disease has inevitably been stimulated by the initial attempts, and this in itself is a useful side-effect. Scadding (1967) in particular felt that 'a somewhat naïve analysis of the meaning of diagnostic statements has been accepted in many studies of the application of computers to diagnosis'. He draws attention to the fact that, 'The mode of operation in (some of) these studies was based upon the most primitive procedure in clinical diagnosis, the Hippocratic method of recognition by similarities of complexes of symptoms and signs to those already described diseases', and hence that, 'Their procedure did not conform to current clinical practice'. His main point appears to be that, 'As knowledge of diseases advances beyond the stage at which they can be defined only on a clinical-descriptive basis, defining characteristics derived from other fields of study are adopted for them'. And, 'Since the exact description of a disease depends upon the defining characteristics we choose to adopt for it, it seems to me possible to think of diseases as not having any sort of independent existence'. The upshot of all this is to demonstrate

> 'that the diagnostic process may end in very different sorts of conclusions; and that the logical and factual implications of

the terms in which these conclusions are expressed differ widely. The "diagnosis" which is the end-point of the process may state no more than the resemblance of the symptoms and signs to a previously recognised pattern; but more usually it makes a statement about aetiology, about a microscopic anatomical abnormality, about a disorder of function, about a specific deficiency or about a biochemical or chromosomal abnormality'.

These comments leave us in no doubt of the ever-increasing complexity of the diagnostic process, as it engages a widening range of disciplines to extend the range of defining characteristics and, hence, the number of identifiable diseases. Identifying a patient as belonging to a particular treatment category is becoming more rather than less information dependent; but there is nothing to support the view that computer-assisted diagnostic procedures are less relevant or even intrinsically more complex. In fact, as the defining characteristics of disease become more dependent on scientific investigation as compared with 'primitive' Hippocratic methods, the computer's task should be easier as the data involved are more precise. It is, however, useful to emphasise the variety of diagnostic conclusions, and remember that data other than that arising from clinical descriptions have commonly to be weighed before arriving at diagnosis; it emphasises the need for medically qualified people to play the dominant role in the design of computer procedures. Scadding also emphasises that in certain cases it may not be possible to demonstrate the defining characteristics at all in living patients, and hence that, 'in such instances a group of observations that can be made clinically, and are relevant to the probability of the presence of the defining characteristic and of the absence of defining characteristics of other diseases, may be selected as diagnostic criteria'. Some care is, therefore, required in the use of the words disease and diagnosis. What is of greater importance however, is; (*a*) that it is the relative specificity of a multiplicity of items of information drawn from clinical-description and other fields of study that determines the likelihood of a particular diagnosis; (*b*) that *some* of these, which is all that are available to the clinician at the early stages of investigation, must prompt the search for the rest; (*c*) that sometimes it is impracticable in a living patient to determine the defining characteristics and, hence, the diagnosis for certain; and (*d*) that a lot of information is involved and is changing, i.e. new knowledge may call for re-definition.

All the more reason then (*a*) that an attempt should be made to structure the disease profiles (including every item-defining characteristic having any relative specificity) together with associated treatment profiles; (*b*) that some organisation should be evolved for overseeing this task as well as for maintaining the validity of these profiles in the light of new knowledge which calls for redefinitions, and for instituting revised weighting factors within the revised definitions. Then, applying the ALF-concept it would, on the basis of the 'Hippocratic phase' of clinical-description, be possible to retrieve from the computer the most likely disease-treatment categories consistent with this evidence *plus* what tests/criteria from other fields of study were required to pursue and identify the defining characteristics. In the event that all tests (short of autopsy) had gone as far as they could towards establishing the defining characteristics, the treatment most justified by the evidence should be adopted. None of this mitigates against the use of the computer; on the contrary, it seems to demand it. By all means drop the phrase computer-assisted diagnosis, if the semantics of the word diagnosis are too confusing, since diagnosis is not the ultimate objective so much as the *action* required. The name, however, is less important than that we should begin to organise and systematise medical knowledge in such a way that it can be stored in computers to facilitate *action*. Academic medicine and medical research may well require a different systematisation orientated according to the logic of conceptual models of disease processes, but the practising clinician does not. He is more directly concerned to relate observed and laboratory test data on a particular patient and to increase the specificity in the direction of the most likely treatment category. As is happening in fields other than medicine, information is becoming action-orientated. It is not so in the medical text books and journals. But, as G. H. Hall has said (Hall, 1967), 'Perhaps in medicine, too, we are due for liberation from the tyranny of words which somehow fail to correspond to our experience, distort our intentions, and fog communications'.

CONVERSATIONAL SYSTEMS: THE TALKING LIBRARY

Over the past 500 years the printed word has been the key element in making the knowledge and experience of others, remote in time and place, available to others. But the rate of discovery is now so fast that words no longer suffice for these purposes. There is now too much print for anyone to cope with; it needs constant research for what is relevant, and often it is obsolete before it is printed. The automatic library facility described earlier indicated at least the possibility of interrogating a library electronically (in which *information* is *suitably organised for the purpose*), which is a major advance in communication capability, especially since it provides access to a single (possibly national) library which it is possible to keep up-to-date. However, since 1964, sufficient progress has been made with the development of remote terminals and computer languages to enable a two-way interchange to take place with the computer-based library. When the first edition of this book was written in 1965, the idea seemed so fanciful that it was not mentioned, and although 'conversational systems' are as yet at an early stage of development it is worth drawing attention to what could well become common practice. The essence of what is involved is best illustrated by Table 1 reproduced from a paper by G. A. Gorry and G. O. Barnett (1968).

Clearly the advice available from such systems can be no better than the quality of the information introduced into the computer programs—and improvement in this depends on the education and training of many more qualified medical personnel. But the process has started ... even among some of the staunchest sceptics of five years ago.

The automatic library facility and the talking library by augmenting the information available to doctors leaves their role essentially unchanged. While this has its advantages, at least in terms of acceptance of computer methods in the initial stages, the future may be very different. Major technological developments, from the steam-engine onwards, have always precipitated radical changes in the organisation of human activity. Given that medicine is the art of the possible, that provided a patient belongs to one or other of the known treatable categories, he is treatable *once the category is identified*, then this latter becomes the initial objective. It could be that history-taking and clinical examination do not turn out to be the most efficient way of making a diagnosis, being too subjective and personalised. It might be that an efficient battery of tests, measurements and questions could be devised

TABLE 1—A Session with the Diagnostic Program*

PLEASE TELL ME ABOUT THE PATIENT
The patient here with me is 23 years old
PLEASE CONTINUE
He shows no evidence of cyanosis
OK PLEASE GO ON
There is no indication of the squatting symptom
ALL RIGHT GO ON PLEASE
I'm afraid that's all I know about him at present
CHECK THE HILAR VESSELS. ARE THEY INCREASED OR DECREASED
They are increased
I SEE
LOOK FOR A LEFT SECOND SYSTOLIC MURMUR
First tell me what the three most probable diseases are at this time
 2 WITH PROBABILITY 74
18 WITH PROBABILITY 7
30 WITH PROBABILITY 3
PLEASE CONTINUE
LOOK FOR A LEFT SECOND SYSTOLIC MURMUR
What is the medical name of disease 2
ATRIAL SEPTAL DEFECT
OK PLEASE GO ON
LOOK FOR A LEFT SECOND SYSTOLIC MURMUR
and the name of disease 18 is
PATENT DUCTUS ARTERIOSUS
ALL RIGHT. GO ON PLEASE
LOOK FOR A LEFT SECOND SYSTOLIC MURMUR
He has a left second midsystolic murmur
ALL RIGHT
IS THE AXIS IN THE ECG RIGHT, LEFT, OR NORMAL
What is the probability of atrial septal defect now
IT IS 94
PLEASE CONTINUE
IS THE AXIS IN THE ECG RIGHT, LEFT, OR NORMAL
It is a right axis
OK
I RECOMMEND A DIAGNOSIS OF DISEASE 2

*User inputs are in lower case letters; program responses are are capital letters.

TABLE 1—*continued*

What is your current view of the problem
MY CURRENT VIEW IS

DISEASE	PROBABILITY
2	93
4	2

Name disease 4 for me
ATRIAL SEPTAL DEFECT WITH PULMONARY HYPER-
  TENSION
I'm finished with this case. Thank you for your help
I HOPE THAT I HAVE BEEN OF SERVICE. GOODBYE

(made possible by scientific progress and economic by automation) to make diagnoses more accurate, not of course at one go, but in a conversational dialogue with a computer-based library accommodating comprehensive and up-to-date medical knowledge. There can be no doubt that this could be achieved to some extent, even on the basis of present knowledge, and progress is likely. It is possible that for a growing range of diagnoses and treatments a doctor may not be needed since a machine with a less-skilled supervisor will do it as well or better (reference chapter One). This will liberate medically qualified manpower for things which new knowledge will make possible (and which, like some modern surgical manoeuvres, require interdisciplinary teams), and for many other things that medicine does inadequately at the present time: disease prevention, epidemiology, attending to psychosomatic disease, the mentally ill, and the aged. Far from being a rash speculation, this would simply follow the well-established pattern already set by machines, enabling a diminishing number of people to do what was done formerly (and this now covers mental as well as muscular activity) and encouraging doctors to create other activities and other types of job. It is most unlikely, therefore, that medicine will be staffed tomorrow as it is today; medicine is now as involved in technological progress as it was for a hundred years wedded to the pace of scientific progress. A final comment from Sir MacFarlane Burnet, writing in the *British Medical Journal* in October 1964, endorses this view.

He writes—

'This raises what may well become the characteristic feature of hospital medicine within the next fifty years, the progressive transfer of decision-making to data-processing machines, or various types of computer. I can see no escape from the contention that if judgement is to be based on experience, then a machine which can give an accurate weight to all the relevant information and express the judgement in terms of a quantitative probability will give a more acceptable answer than any clinician.'

And later on in the same article,

'. . . there will be need of men who are much more mathematicians and biochemists than physicians, in our present sense of the term, but who will also need to apply common sense, courage and compassion in handling all the human difficulties that escape the machines.'

REFERENCES

Gorry, G. A. and Barnett, G. O. (1968) Sequential diagnosis by computer. *Journal of the American Medical Association*, 205, 12.
Hall, G. H. (1967) Letter to *Lancet*, ii, 984.
Scadding, J. G. (1967) Diagnosis: the clinician and the computer. *Lancet*, ii, 877.

8
Computer-assisted Measurement, Analysis and Communication

CHARACTER CHANGES INDUCED BY SCIENTIFIC PROGRESS

THE SUSTAINED AND GROWING IMPACT of scientific progress on medicine can best be described by way of an anecdote. A man with a beard from which one hair has been extracted is asked the question, 'do you still have a beard', to which, of course, he gives an affirmative answer. A second hair is extracted and the question gives rise to a similar answer. One hair at a time the procedure is repeated until there comes a stage when the man's answer changes and he decides that maybe he no longer has a beard. A step-wise change in character has been induced, yet at no stage was the situation significantly different from before. Many examples of this phenomenon abound in our society. A step-wise change in the character of commuting has been caused by adding just a few more passengers a day; a step-wise change in the character of our towns and cities has been produced by adding just a few more cars each day; a step-wise change in the character of certain residential areas has been induced by adding just a few more coloured immigrants a week; a step-wise change in the fortunes of local grocers and newsagents has been induced by just a few more supermarkets a month; a step-wise change in the character of our postmen, policemen, teachers and even doctors has been induced by the one-hair-at-a-time inflationary pressures eroding real remuneration levels in their state-controlled activities. Every Minister can honestly argue that things are not significantly different from when he took office but . . . one-hair-at-a-time . . . step-wise changes in character are induced, which very often would provoke the strongest reactions if they were more localised in time. This is relevant here as it draws attention to the step-wise changes in character of medical practice induced by the one-hair-at-a-time introduction of scientific measurement, which now require step-wise changes in organisation and facilities of the health services to cope with the new and changed situation. Not so long ago, certainly within the living memory of older doctors, the stethoscope, the thermometer, the sphygmomanometer, the ophthalmoscope, and occasionally the electrocardiograph, together with a capacity and training for observation of symptoms and signs, provided adequate equipment for resolving most diagnostic situations*. But scientific progress has greatly extended the range of precision of human perception: a wide variety of measurements of otherwise unobservable phenomena now add significantly to the information available for patient management. Commonly such measurements call for the use of specialised equipment and laboratory procedures, and the associated service departments with their special skills are the fastest growing part of the modern hospital environment. In the case of biochemical laboratories, for example, the workload is doubling about every four or five years and has been doing so for over two decades.

Three important consequences follow. First, the individual clinician or surgeon no longer makes all the detailed observations on which the success of his diagnosis or treatment depends; he must rely on the competence of others. Secondly, there arises an acute communication problem involving language and identification difficulties, as well as delays and inaccuracies. Thirdly, the rate of dependence of medicine on measurement is pushing up the workload of the service units so fast (thousands of tests a week are now quite common) that the administration, production and checking of results can no longer be dealt with by the informal methods of the scientific backroom, but require business-like procedures to ensure all round efficiency, both in respect of the accuracy, speed and cost of the results produced and in the handling of the associated paper work. These consequences amount to a step-wise change in character requiring corresponding changes in organisation and facilities; fortunately, the advent of the new data technology is timely in this respect, since its efficient deployment reinforces the need for changes in organisation.

*Those who complacently think it is still so should look at the results of any of the multiphasic screening exercises that have been undertaken in recent years: what the eye does not see . . . .

An Example: The Biochemical Laboratory

All these features are well exemplified in the growth of mechanisation in the biochemical laboratory. One of the earliest tests was to estimate the level of glucose in the blood, as part of the management of diabetes, made possible by the discovery of insulin in the 1920s. Subsequently, with the development of micro-methods, it became possible to estimate a number of constituents from very small blood samples, which measurably contributed to the diagnosis of metabolic disorders. And with the introduction of the flame photometer to measure sodium and potassium levels in body fluids, the workload of biochemical laboratories steadily increased.

A major advance in coping with the rising demand came with the invention in 1957 by Skeggs, in America, of continuous flow analytical equipment which was developed and marketed under the proprietary label 'Auto-Analyzer' (Plate 7B). Essentially, it consists of a revolving tray which holds the patients' specimens in a series of cups; these are sequentially sampled, separated by an air gap, and pumped through tubes; reagents, as appropriate, are added on the way and after measurements by a colorimeter, or flame photometer the results are presented as a series of peaks on a continuous pen-recorder chart (Plate 8A). The overall effect of this mechanisation of 'wet bench methods' has been to increase the output per technician by some 300 per cent to around 18,000 tests per technician-year.

At the same time, of course, it is necessary to organise workloads for the machines, and to cope with the results at the rate they are produced, as well as to implement active procedures for quality control to ensure the validity of the results. This is precisely where automatic data-processing and automation are relevant.

Considerable experience has now been acquired from some 25 biochemical laboratories in the U.K. which have been using computers in various ways, some for nearly ten years. It is still true to say that there is no single universally accepted computer laboratory system.

It is appropriate to go into this application in some detail since it illustrates many of the difficulties and characteristics inherent in the business of using computers.

As has already been explained there existed an ever-increasing workload which was threatening to swamp bigger laboratories. The need to change and mechanise methods grew yearly more urgent. It has taken several years, however, to establish some concensus among biochemists and pathologists as to what was required. Little experience of using computers existed. A period of trial and error was inevitable, hence the diversity of operation during the first twenty or so installations. The difficulty of establishing a generally acceptable method is a very real one to to the supplier of such equipment. It is unrealistic to expect a manufacturer to supply a specially developed system tailored to each user; some common basis has to be developed to make the investment viable. Moreover, the potential user cannot afford to pay the cost of a specially developed one-off system. This is a recurring problem with all computer applications in every field. There has to be a consensus among users in order to establish a market. And there has to be a realisation that installing a computer is likely to lead to a complete reorganisation of the laboratory.

Secondly, the application illustrates the development from 'off-line' to 'on-line' methods. In the 'off-line' method, data are collected from the instruments and converted to a medium suitable for input to a computer and then taken to the computer for processing, the results being sent back to the pathologist for entry into reports. There are various ways of taking signals from laboratory instruments and presenting the computer with a digitised result on paper tape. This is not the place to go into this process in detail. Suffice it to say that any mechanised method that is simple and not too costly is better than any manual method that relies on human observation of readings and their subsequent recalibration and correction by human calculation.

Biochemists were quick to appreciate that in using the computer for calculation it would not be difficult to develop programs so that all results could be checked by statistical method, which would bring a new level of quality control into laboratories. Quality control of results also allowed the biochemist to know how the instruments themselves were behaving.

Accuracy, throughput and quality control could all be even further improved if the instruments could be tapped directly and the signal (a voltage) put straight into the computer system. If this could be practically achieved a dynamic method of controlling the process could be evolved. Thus arose the demand for 'on-line' methods; where the computer system is part of the laboratory instrument system and actually controls the instrument performance (Whitehead, 1969).

A computer system can also enable the pathologist to refer to the patient's previous record and to compare the current result with these previous results. The ability to use cumulative records is not strictly confined to computer systems, off-line or on-line. The fact is that to store and retrieve patient pathology records is so cumbersome by manual methods that it is never effectively done except where magnetic discs are available on a computer system.

Thirdly, it has to be appreciated that in depending on a semi-automated system in the biochemistry laboratory part of the clinical management of the patient becomes dependent on machine performance. A pathology laboratory is a service laboratory; it is not a research laboratory where machine breakdown is, rarely, calamitous. Reliability of hardware, of software and of system performance is absolutely fundamental. The system must be simple and there must be an established and easily worked fall-back system when the inevitable mechanical breakdown occurs. Electrical circuitry is now generally highly reliable, but no machine (or human for that matter) can perform to 100 per cent reliability. This fact must be squarely faced.

Fourthly, any computer system must be flexible. It must be capable of taking on new instruments as they come into use and new laboratories as they need computerisation. It must be capable of adding laboratories near at hand or at distant points, using the Post Office transmission lines. Such flexibility calls for a close link between the computer and communications systems. This is an increasingly important fact in every computer system as we pointed out in chapter 5. Indeed, the association of computing power and communications is the likely big development in computer application over the next decade. What is required is a system the basic elements of which can be used in any laboratory. Special software need be developed only to fit the basic system to each laboratory. As more and more laboratories use the basic system then more varying special software is available. This software is usually referred to as Application Software. Each successive laboratory using a basic pathology computer system

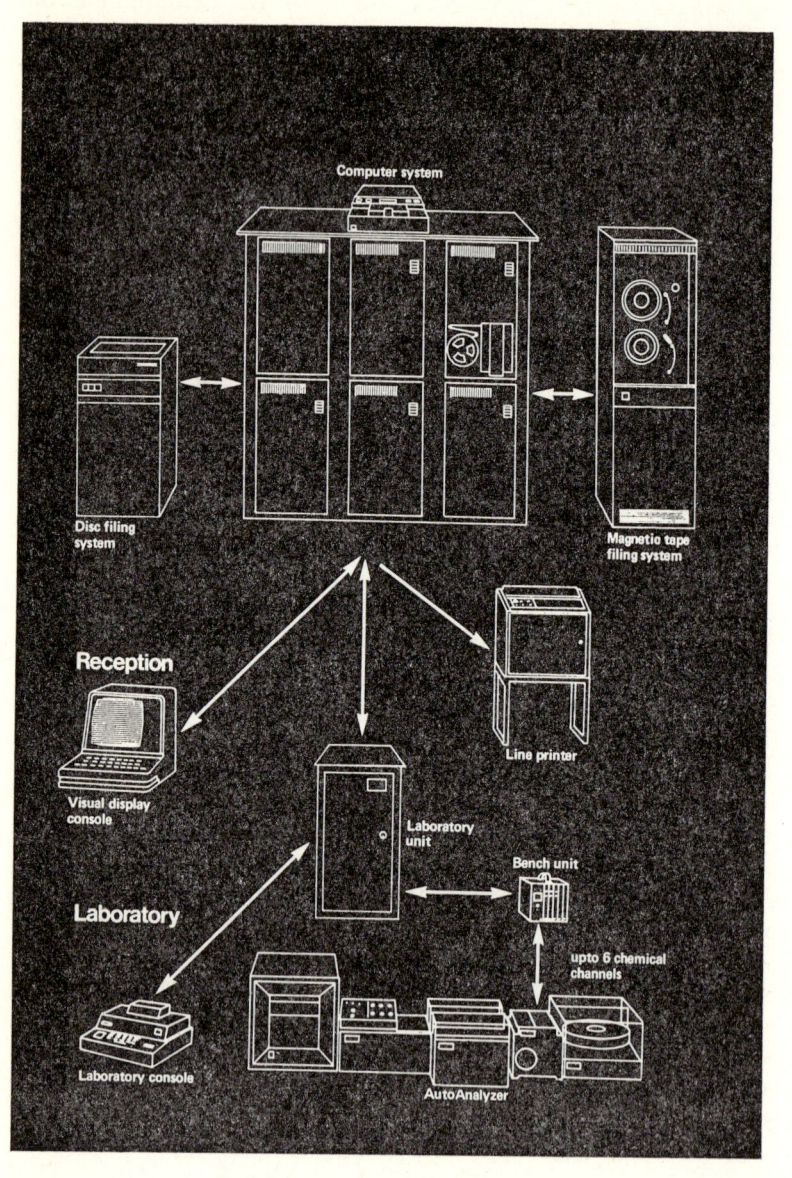

Figure 5. A typical Pathlab system

will find more application programs already developed to choose from.

Under the sponsorship of the Department of Health and Social Security the current situation in the U.K. is the beginning of the establishment of such a basic system.

The fifth point that applying computers to pathology has illustrated is that the development of any system never turns out to be as simple as was originally thought, nor as exciting, and often the emphasis changes during development. In the mid-sixties the problem was the acquisition of data from instruments and how best to do this. In fact, experience has shown that the problem of processing the request forms and of delivering results and reports on time to the clinician making the request is a much more difficult procedure to computerise, requiring, as it does, complete reorganisation. The development of any system is a long, tedious business, demanding persistence, and costing much more than would be suspected. Every detail has to be right.

There are many other points about the use of computers in pathology laboratories that are of more interest to biochemists and pathologists than the general reader. Within the next few years we can expect to see every district hospital and most GPs in the United Kingdom served by a laboratory which is dependent on a computer. A typical Pathlab system is illustrated schematically in Figure 5.

PATIENT MONITORING

Cardiology Departments in hospitals have much instrumentation for monitoring patients at risk. Indeed, it is an obvious fact that throughout the hospital instrumentation is proliferating.

A number of experimental and research applications in the use of computers in controlling such instrumentation have been attempted, chiefly in the U.S.A. None has become an established method and many problems connected with signal noise level, patient discomfort, cost and presentation of results remain unresolved.

A system exists in America in which computers are used to diagnose ECG results centrally. ECG data are input from a wide area, expert interpretation is made and results output to the peripheral point.

PATTERN RECOGNITION

Much diagnostic information from graphical and digital data becomes significant to an experienced observer by recognition of patterns of trends, for example the interpretation of X-rays.

Interesting philosophical problems of definition arise in any attempt to systematise pattern recognition by using computers. The major medical experiment currently being conducted in the U.K. to research into pattern recognition is at the M.R.C. Population and Clinical Cytogenetic Unit in the Western General Hospital in Edinburgh. Dr D. Rutovitz is using a multi-processor system of small computers to establish a machine method of recognising chromosome patterns. Normally, this is done by particularly laborious manual methods. If large numbers of chromosome patterns are to be observed it is essential to use machine methods. The outcome is still to be determined.

Similar methods have been used to investigate the possibility of using computers in cytological screening of cervical smears.

RADIATION TREATMENT PLANNING

One of the first useful applications of computers to medicine was in radiation treatment planning, where the objective is to administer a lethal dose of radiation to malignant tissues while minimising the dosage to non-malignant regions. This is usually accomplished by using multiple radiation sources so placed that their intersections (where their respective contributions summate) are located in the area of the malignant tissue ('multiple field therapy'); alternatively, a single source is rotated about an axis to produce a similar effect ('rotational therapy'); or small radioactive sources such as needles or tubes are inserted at strategic positions in and around the malignant tissue ('interstitial therapy').

In every case the problem of calculating the radiation dosage distribution can be reduced to calculating the dose at a single point from a single radiation source. If this is repeated for each of the radiation sources involved, addition will give the total dose at a single point. If repeated for all points on a co-planar grid of suitable mesh-size it gives the total dosage in a plane and if repeated for parallel planes at some suitable interval it gives the total dosage distribution throughout any specified volume. Distributions throughout sub-volumes and sub-planes and at discrete points are similarly dealt with by specifying the appropriate boundary points. For this reason a general-purpose computer program for radiation treatment planning need make no fundamental distinction between multiple-field, rotational and interstitial therapies, the essential difference between them being the radiation pattern characterising each source involved, and the various positions in which they are deployed.

One of the commonest ways of calculating the dose at a single point without computers is by using isodose charts, each of which in effect represents graphically the radiation pattern of each type and strength of source used. An isodose chart is so constructed

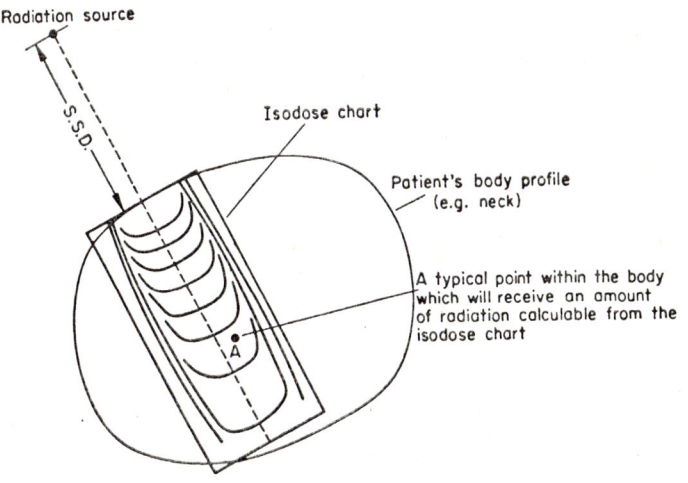

Figure 6. Overlaying an isodose chart

(there are mathematical and empirical methods for doing this) that it corresponds to the dosage distribution for a particular source placed a certain distance from the body—usually called the source-to-skin distance (SSD). When evaluating the dosage distribution manually the chart is overlaid on the body profile and the dosage at a point A (Figure 6) is interpolated between the contours on the isodose chart, corrections being applied to allow for such things as oblique fields, air gaps, tissue excesses and field weighting factors. This is repeated for all points of interest, and for each radiation source involved.

To computerise this procedure the isodose chart must be

digitised (usually expressed as a grid of points) and stored in the computer. To do this accurately may involve more than a thousand sets of co-ordinates per isodose chart, of which there may be several hundred. The inconvenience of preparing and inserting this amount of data may be avoided by using one of a number of methods which enable the computer itself to generate the equivalent of the isodose chart data from considerably less data by means of suitable formulae or algorithms. The computer is equally helpful in preparing and outputting the data: it can, for example, express the dosage at every single point as a percentage of the maximum dose, or, as is often required, as a percentage of the modal dose (i.e. that most frequently occurring in the malignant region). Most useful of all it can interpolate the contours of constant dosage, so as to enable a graph-plotting machine to produce an easily assimilable map of the radiation dosage distribution.

The operating procedure itself is fairly straightforward. Data specifying the patient's body outline (neck, abdomen, and so on), the positions at which the various radiation sources are to be placed, the isodose charts to be used, any field weighting factors, as well as the type of output (numerical, graphical) required, are systematically set out on a checkable pro forma, and telephoned, teleprinted or (if time allows) simply posted to a computer centre, where after punching they are inserted into the computer. The radiation dosage distribution will be evaluated quickly and accurately and at little cost, and the results either directly printed out (or automatically drawn out for a contoured presentation) or generated in the form of punched paper tape so that they can be teleprinted back for local printing or graph-plotting on off-line equipment.

With the introduction of terminals and VDUs the operating procedure can be significantly improved. The data are inserted locally via a terminal keyboard, and within a matter of minutes (depending on the complexity of the treatment plan involved) the contoured dosage distribution will appear on a graphic display. The radiotherapist can then, if he chooses, key-in altered values for field sizes, positions and angles, and quickly obtain a revised treatment plan; this enables optimisation by successive calculation to be accomplished effortlessly to a level that is simply not a practical proposition by manual methods because of the time and skill required. In fact, with computer-assisted radiation treatment planning, the only limit to a fully optimal plan is that determined by the quality of the basic data, rather than by the time and skill available, and this is providing an incentive to overcome these limitations. Indeed, as confidence and facility increase, thought is now being given to how the computer may assist in deciding the initial choice of radiation source configuration to provide a specified dosage distribution, hitherto a combination of experience and reference to similar previous plans. Some useful progress has already been made in this area. Once again the logic of these developments is tending towards specialised units developing useful computer programs to service major areas. Trained cerebral activity of the type that can evaluate a plan to meet a radiotherapist's dosage specification will no longer be needed in every local unit; the best of it will combine to produce high-grade computer-assisted facilities of wide utility, and the rest will be displaced to other tasks. The result should be greater productivity per unit of trained cerebral effort, greater accuracy and better treatment, known operating standards (in place of individual variety), a speedier and more direct service for the radiotherapist, and more concentrated research on improved methods.

MEDICAL RESEARCH

Measurement, analysis, and especially mathematical and statistical calculation, are at the root of all scientific activity, and so not surprisingly the bio-medical sciences were among the first to use computers in varied calculations. More recently, computers have entered the laboratories themselves to control instruments, filter off unwanted data, interpret data and present it in a variety of ways, so that trends and patterns are visually assimilable, enabling the researcher to interact on-line with his experimental work.

Perhaps the most conspicuous example of all is the way in which computers have contributed to the spectacular progress of molecular biology, which is within promise of extending the threshold capability of therapeutics. The basic technique, devices by Perutz, involves the replacing of various atoms in crystallised protein molecules by heavier metal atoms to provide stronger reference points, scanning them by an X-ray beam to obtain diffraction pictures resulting from the beam's electron-scattering effects, and from these pictures deducing the relative electron densities and positions of the atoms in the crystal by means of monumental calculations. Many aspects of this technique lend themselves to automation of the sort described in this chapter and as a result the computer-assisted procedures provide a powerful tool in the analysis of proteins and other living substances.

Following the first major phase of molecular biology, which concluded with the unravelling of the genetic code found chemically in the double-helical structure of deoxyribonucleic acid (DNA), the emphasis has now shifted outwards from the cell nucleus to the rest of the cell; and far from being undifferentiated protoplasm as was previously thought, molecular biology assisted by the electron microscope has shown it to be a highly organised array of structures known collectively as organelles, the seat of many different enzyme systems. It is these enzymes, now being systematically identified by automated X-ray diffraction methods, which are likely to lead to major advances in therapeutics. Enzymes, too, are proteins, and in their dynamic role as catalysts in biochemical reactions, it would appear that they mediate every living process from breathing and digestion to basic thought mechanisms. So far about a thousand different enzymes have been identified. The first of these to have its structure fully elucidated was lysozyme, its precise atomic structure being the outcome of a five-year effort by Dr D. C. Phillips and his colleagues at the Royal Institution, London. Since then, despite the enormous complexity of these structures, various groups on both sides of the Atlantic have managed, with better computers and more automated procedures, to determine the structure of a dozen or so enzymes, and it is likely that progress will accelerate.

Medical Research covers a wide filed of activity. Many examples of the use of computers to aid medical research could be given in animal experiment control, in biology, in psychology, in cytology, and so on. In nearly every case the computer is being used to aid quantitative measurement—as a calculator. In several instances the use of computers has enabled more accurate control of the experiment and more detailed calculation or correlation of results. These examples are specialised applications and their significance is probably only appreciated by someone involved in the particular research. When straight calculation capability is required, access can often be obtained to university computers, although the M.R.C. runs a central computer unit to provide this service to its units.

SIMULATION: MODELLING PROCESSES

Another important use of computers, independent of their use in processing paper-work, making calculations, interpreting data from instruments, and presenting results in a variety of ways, is in providing simulation facilities.

The purpose of simulation is to examine the workings of a particular set of assumptions or relationships as they pertain to a situation which is either too risky, or too costly or too time-consuming to examine directly. Model aircraft are 'flown' in wind tunnels, model ships are sailed in large water-tanks; tidal flows are modelled in miniature, and so on, so that the limits of operating performance can be ascertained. The essential requirement is to make the model (the 'analogue') of the true situation realistic in all relevant aspects so that reasonably valid inferences may be drawn about the true situation.

Physical analogues such as models of ships and aircraft need no explanation. But in some situations, such as weather forecasting or determining cardiopulmonary function, it is intrinsically more difficult to devise physical analogues; instead, mathematical equations are used. The selected formulae describe the processes involved well enough to enable valid inferences to be drawn, as for example, when equations of gas exchange in the cardiopulmonary system enable inferences to be drawn about the respiratory, circulatory and metabolic responses of patients to various levels of exercise. The mathematical equations in these cases form *abstract* analogues (rather than physical analogues) of the situations being examined. Useful mathematical analogues (or mathematical models as they are sometimes called) have been devised for a whole variety of situations ranging from missile trajectories and the spread of epidemics to many different types of bodily function (renal, neural, optical, circulatory, and so on). Special machines have been constructed for carrying out the kinds of mathematical equations involved, hence the name 'analogue computers'. Analogue computers have existed in one form or another since 1930; essentially they are calculators but when, for example, they are performing calculations that relate to the cardiopulmonary system they are said to be analogues (or mathematical models) of the cardiopulmonary system, and so on.

All well and good, but it is a matter of fact that only a very small part, perhaps less than one per cent, of our universe of activity and experience can be formulated in mathematical terms. This is one of the severe limitations of mathematics; it is also the reason why most people for most of the time get on very well without them. On the other hand, a great deal of what each of us does exhibits some degree of order and systematisation. Our professional activity may vary from day to day, a patient may differ in his individual response, but it is not unique; we are continually recognising similar circumstances to which we tend to respond similarly, whatever our particular activity. Were it not so, were our lives not substantially regulated and ordered, there would be little chance of consolidating our experience. We should be improvising from scratch every time, and experience and professionalism would count for nought. Just one simple and familiar example: any intelligent driver who regularly commutes during the rush-hour will have learned to optimise his journey-time by allowing for the incidence of traffic at various points on route. This does not take the form of a mathematical calculation, because no relevant formula of wide generality applies, nevertheless it is typical of many practical situations in that it admits of intelligent scrutiny and rationalisation.

By contrast with that very tiny part of natural knowledge that can be accurately described in mathematical terms, the part which can be intelligently described and pursued, and which bears ordered resemblance to what has gone before, is largely predictable and manageable in terms of response and makes up the greater part of what we do. It is this vast area of activity and experience that can be modelled on the modern digital computer. As was indicated in the first chapter, digital computers have liberated us from mathematics; they enable us for the first time to model and explore processes and behaviour (e.g. traffic situations) exhibiting much looser logical organisation than that to which the more stringent logical frameworks of mathematics and statistics are applicable.

Such is the versatility of data technology that sets of rules (algorithms) can be used for model-making in place of mathematical formulae. Models can thus be designed to generate actual arterial blood-pressure curves, actual electrocardiographic traces, rather than mathematical idealisations of them, if it will enhance their realism for any purpose. This, once computer competence is more widespread, should make simulation far more generally useful than it has been to date; in testing and predicting the effect of operative chemotherapeutic and anaesthetic procedures for example, in simulating the effect of an additional operating theatre or intensive care unit or in changed staffing procedures in existing ones. Realistic simulation should enable guess-work based on experience to be refined. Everyone has had their laughs at the so-called war games and business games, but the value of these in exercising responses to realistic situations has greatly increased with the increasing realism of the simulation. Any expensive or risky manoeuvre is worth simulating realistically to determine its shortcomings *before* it is embarked upon, and this refinement of planning and management decisions is inevitable. Simulation therefore is as useful in refining existing activity or evaluating proposed changes in activity as it is in testing the validity of hypotheses in research work.

To point the way to what is possible, we might consider the simulation possibilities of the ALF-procedure in exercising students in their diagnostic roles. From the disease-treatment directory stored in the computer, it would be possible to select items of data and so present a simulated patient exhibiting particular signs and symptoms. This might be done by print-out in the simplest case, but there is no reason why the disease-treatment directory should not be augmented by pictures of patients at particular stages of each disease-process so that the patient could be presented visually on a display. The student would be invited to write down his views on the differential diagnosis, together with a proposed course of action. Once this was done he could key in the relevant data to the computer and request its views on the differential diagnosis and action to be taken (in this capacity the computer would be carrying out the ALF-procedure). Given this additional information, the student would finally decide his course of action and key it into the computer. The computer, now acting in the role of simulator, could determine from its stored information the effect of this action on the patient, and so display the result. The interaction described would be repeated until the student gave up or had arrived at his own firm conclusion. In either case he would then request all the information on the patient including diagnosis and treatment. There would be obvious satisfaction in the case of being right, but also satisfaction in the case of being wrong—at least to the extent of knowing that only a simulated patient was at risk!

It has been possible in this chapter only to indicate some of the principal features of automated measurement and analysis, with some examples that point out the operating principles involved. Computers are increasingly being used in many dedicated applications, as we have indicated. It is our hope that the explanations we have offered will arouse the general interest of the reader sufficiently for him (or her) to want to examine any computer project that is being conducted within his own or an adjacent medical organisation. If he understands the general background of the computer aspects of the project his own medical knowledge will combine with this to allow a ready appreciation of the significance of the project and its possible application to his own specialty. Ample technical literature exists for more detailed study of computer technology, for which the British Computer Society will be able to give references.

REFERENCE

Whitehead, T. P. ed. (1969) Automation and data processing in pathology. *Journal of Clinical Pathology*, **22**, Supplement 3.

Appendix 1
How the Computer Works

ALTHOUGH MOST of what people need to know about computers has already been dealt with in previous chapters, many people are curious to know how a data-procedure is actually carried out under program control, that is how the central processor works. This appendix is an attempt to satisfy that curiosity.

Inevitably it is rather tedious because computers themselves are tedious. A computer is capable of performing only a dozen or so elementary operations and any particular procedure that it is desired to carry out must first be analysed into a sequence of such elementary operations (programming). Once this is done, however, the sole virtue of the machine is its ability to carry out such sequences of elementary operations at a rate of about a million a second.

A CENTRAL PROCESSOR

To explain how a central processor works requires us first to explain in detail a typical set of elementary operations; second to show how they are interconnected in a central processor; and last to explain how they can be operated under program control. Neither special background knowledge nor exceptional intelligence are necessary to follow and understand these explanations but it does require the capacity to follow a few pages of boring detail, at the end of which one can join the magic circle of the initiates and their esoteric incantations.

A typical set of elementary computer operations is shown in Figure 7. The addition operation represented by the code 0 is such that if two numbers a and b are contained in two registers*

*A register is simply a physical device, such as a keyboard or a ferrite core store (to be explained) which stores a number or a word.

connected to a box 0, then it produces the result $a + b$ in another register; the subtraction operation, code 1, similarly produces $a - b$; the clear operation, code 2, is such that if a register contains any number a, then by circulating it through box 2 it clears the register, i.e. leaves zero in it. The left shift operation, code 3, is such that if a register contains any number a and it is passed through box 3, then the number is 'left-shifted' one decimal place, i.e. 49 becomes 490; left shift is thus equivalent to multiplication

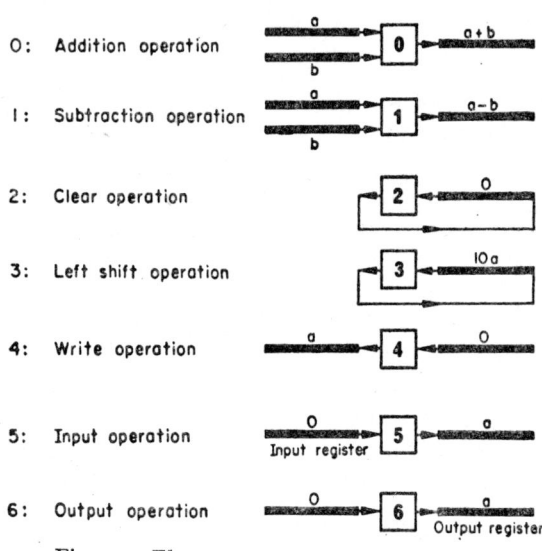

0:	Addition operation	
1:	Subtraction operation	
2:	Clear operation	
3:	Left shift operation	
4:	Write operation	
5:	Input operation	
6:	Output operation	

Figure 7. Elementary computer operations

by 10. The 'write' operation, code 4, is such that any number a in the register on the right is transferred to the register on the left, leaving zero in the register on the right. The input operation, code 5, transfers any number a from the so-called 'input register' on the left to the register on the right of box 5; the output operation, code 6, transfers any number a from the register on the left to the 'output register' on the right of box 6; boxes 4, 5 and 6 in fact perform very similar operations: they all simply transfer a number.

The details of these boxes need not bother us; suffice it that each one performs some elementary operation which it is very easy to design. The interesting and surprising thing is that these opera-

Appendix 1 117

tions alone are sufficient to make up a very realistic computer. Figure 8 shows how they are connected together. The main feature of this organisation is that all boxes are joined to a special register called the accumulator, and, where appropriate, the

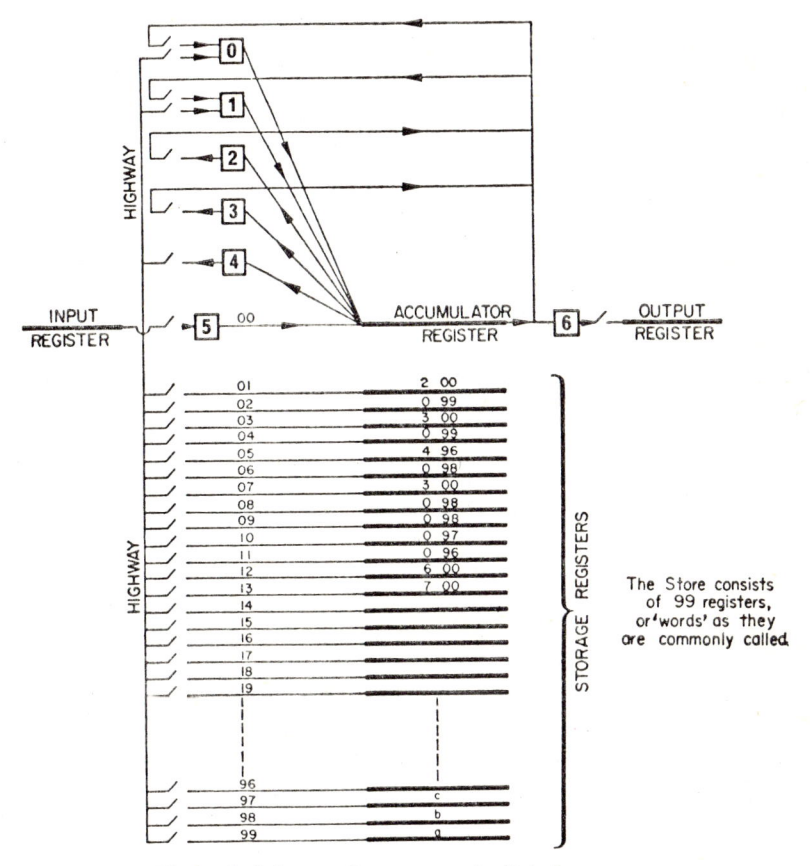

Figure 8. Schema of an automatic digital computer

boxes can be connected to any of 99 registers (or 'words' as they are commonly called) comprising the store, by closing switches. The number of each register is called its 'address'; the accumulator has the address 00.

The *modus operandi* of this particular configuration (which is the way all central processors are organised) can be seen by supposing that the accumulator contains *a*, and that the register 98 contains *b* (the other numbers shown in the registers in Figure 8 should be ignored for the moment). Closing the switches 0 and 98 (written 0 98) joins the accumulator register and register 98 to box 0, and as a result $a + b$ is left in the accumulator; thus, it will be seen that by closing the switches 0 and that of any storage register, the contents of that storage register are added into the accumulator. 0 is therefore called the addition operation. In a similar way 1 98 (i.e. closing the switches 1 and 98) leaves $a - b$ in the accumulator and 1 is called the subtraction operation. 2 00, i.e. closing the switch 2, circulates the number in the accumulator through box 2, thus leaving zero in the accumulator; operation 2 is therefore called the clear operation. 3 00, i.e. closing switch 3, circulates the number in the accumulator through box 3 thus leaving 10*a* in the accumulator; operation 3 is therefore called the left-shift operation. 4 96, i.e. closing the switches 4 and 96, joins the accumulator to box 4 and on to register 96, thus causing the number *a* in the accumulator to be 'written' or transferred to register 96, leaving zero in the accumulator; 4 is called the write operation. 5 00, i.e. closing switch 5, causes whatever number is in the input register, *a* say, to be transferred to the accumulator; 5 is thus called the input operation. 6 00, i.e. closing switch 6, causes the number *a* in the accumulator to be transferred to the output register, leaving the accumulator zero; 6 is called the output operation.

A mechanism of this sort has something in common with a piano. Just as a supplier of pianos might reasonably say to a purchaser, 'you can play any tune whatsoever on it', while perhaps omitting the crux of the problem, 'provided you press the keys in the right sequence', so a computer supplier might say to a purchaser, 'you can perform any data-procedure whatsoever on that', while failing to mention the crux of the problem, 'provided you close the switches in the right sequence'. The composition, or the program, as we shall see is everything. Well, just as one might doodle on a piano keyboard on one's first encounter with it, let us as-it-were doodle on the switches of our central processor mechanism and see what happens. It will be supposed that register 99, 98 and 97 respectively contain the numbers *a*, *b* and *c*, and that the following sequence of twelve switches is activated, in turn—

Switching Sequence (or program)		Description of What Happens (accumulator contents after each operation)
1.	2 00	0
2.	0 99	a
3.	3 00	$10a$
4.	0 99	$11a$
5.	4 96	0 (register 96 now contains $11a$)
6.	0 98	b
7.	3 00	$10b$
8.	0 98	$11b$
9.	0 98	$12b$
10.	0 97	$12b + c$
11.	0 96	$11a + 12b + c$
12.	6 00	0 ($11a + 12b + c$ is transferred to the output register)

The first instruction 2 00 clears the accumulator; the second instruction 0 99 adds the contents of register 99, namely a, to the accumulator contents, thus leaving $a + 0$, or simply a in the accumulator; the third instruction 3 00 left shifts the contents of the accumulator which as a result contains $10a$; the fourth instruction 0 99 adds the contents of register 99 to the accumulator which thus contains $11a$; the fifth instruction 4 96 writes the contents of the accumulator into register 96, leaving the accumulator zero; the sixth instruction 0 98 adds the contents of register 98 to the accumulator, which as a result contains b; the seventh instruction 3 00 left shifts the accumulator, which as a result contains $10b$; the eighth and ninth instructions, both 0 98, add the contents of register 98 to the accumulator twice, which as a result contains $12b$; the tenth instruction 0 97 adds the contents of register 97 to the accumulator, which thus contains $12b + c$; the eleventh instruction adds the contents of register 96 to the accumulator which as a result contains $11a + 12b + c$; finally, the twelfth instruction 6 00 transfers the accumulator contents to the output register, leaving the accumulator zero.

If the reader has followed the last few pages carefully he will have grasped a fundamental point, namely that if the *switching sequence* specified by the twelve numbers is executed, then the formula $11a + 12b + c$ will have been *calculated* from the three numbers a, b and c. A different switching sequence would give rise to a different calculation; and, conversely, to perform a particular calculation one must determine the appropriate switching sequence. Clearly, the same sequence of twelve numbers just described would calculate the quantity $11a + 12b + c$ for *any* three numbers a, b and c placed in registers 99, 98 and 97; the same sequence can therefore be repeated on different sets of data. For example, if we had determined a sequence of numbers for evaluating income tax, then the same sequence could be applied to different individual's salaries in turn. It does not matter therefore that it may take a long time to determine the right sequence (quicker methods are discussed later) because once determined the sequence can be used again and again.

THE STORED PROGRAM

The sequence of twelve numbers in the above example is called a '*program*', each individual number being called an '*instruction*' (or sometimes an '*order*'). The complete sequence is written as a list of numbers and called a 'program of instructions'. It will be noted that the first digit of every instruction specifies an elementary computer operation, and is usually called the '*function part*' of the instruction, whereas the last two digits specify the address of a register, and so are called the '*address part*' of the instruction.

Example: instruction   4   96

                               ↗   ↖

               function part   address part

    Thus, any calculation (and as will be seen later on, any procedure involving alphabetical data) can be expressed or '*programmed*' as a sequence of elementary computer operations provided by the computer designer. Different computers vary somewhat in the basic operations available, and each uses its own particular codes for each elementary operation but as will be seen later, there is now a marked tendency towards adopting similar conventions in all machines.

    The fact that a program can be written down as a list of numbers is of the utmost importance, for it means that *the program itself can be stored inside the computer* along with the data. In the example above, the twelve numbers constituting the program could be stored in registers 01 to 12 as shown in Figure 9. This is

Appendix 1 121

exactly what is done in practice, and on pressing the start-button a control unit (not shown in the figure) starting with the first register 01, takes each number (or instruction) in turn, separately decodes the function digit and address digits, and closes the switches automatically. Because the mechanism for doing this is

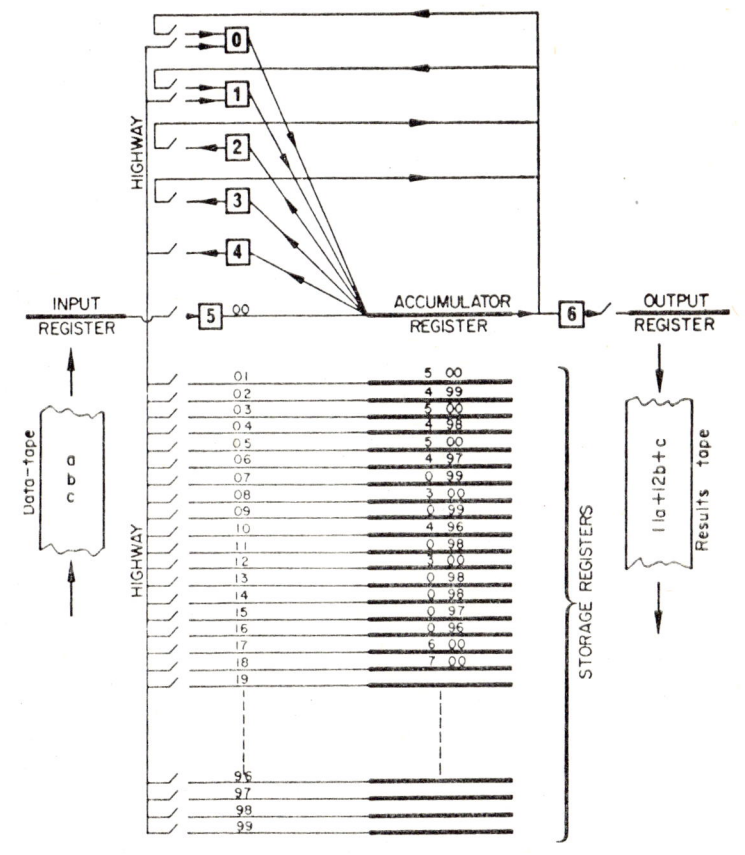

Figure 9. Schema showing stored program, data-tape and results-tape

wholly electronic these actions take place incredibly quickly, the twelve instructions being completed in less than 1/10,000 of a second. Computer speeds vary, each instruction taking between a ten-thousandth and a millionth of a second to be obeyed, depending on the cost of the computer. The control unit must have some means of knowing when the last instruction has been reached, and this is achieved by ending each program with 7 00, the 'stop' instruction which, when decoded by the control unit, stops the mechanism. (The manner in which a control unit decodes each number and closes the corresponding switches is similar to the techniques used by the Post Office for decoding and switching telephone numbers; it need not concern us here.)

The essential nature of automatic digital computing and of programming should be evident from the last few pages. Data and program are inserted into the computer store (in a way shortly to be described), and on pressing the start-button the control causes each instruction to be obeyed, in turn, until it meets the last instruction, which stops the machine; by this time the final result will be in the output register which usually drives an automatic teleprinter. No manual intervention is involved from the time the start-button is pressed to when the results are ejected from the computer. In a sense, it could be said that 'the computer is calculating the formula', and if the calculation it was performing corresponded to that for a missile trajectory, or a weather forecast, or a radiation treatment plan, then it could indeed be said that the computer was 'doing' these things. In fact, however, it is just carrying out slavishly and step-by-step the sequence of instructions that have been programmed for it; it is merely carrying out what it has been ordered to perform, and if the sequence of instructions has any practical significance, it will only be what has been invested in it by the program designer.

The reader may like to follow through the two programs on p. 123, or better still, construct them independently, and compare. If he does so he may find that his program is slightly different; this does not mean necessarily that it is wrong, since different sequences of instructions may fulfil the same purpose, i.e. programs are not unique.

Every calculation and data-procedure to be executed by a computer *must* at some stage be broken down into this degree of detail, in which each instruction in code form specifies a particular elementary operation of the machine. This is what is known as programming in *machine code*—a code directly related to the elementary computer operations. It is a very tedious business, and happily, computer scientists have devised so-called *high-level* languages which obviate the need for writing programs directly in machine code form, thus enabling a form of pidgin English to

(a) Calculate $8a + b - c$

Program		Description
1.	2 00	Clear Accumulator
2.	0 99	Acc. contains a
3.	3 00	,, ,, $10a$
4.	1 99	,, ,, $9a$
5.	1 99	,, ,, $8a$
6.	0 98	,, ,, $8a+b$
7.	1 97	,, ,, $8a+b-c$
8.	6 00	Output $8a+b-c$
9.	7 00	Stop

(b) Calculate $a + 9b - 9c$

Program		Description
1.	2 00	Clear Accumulator
2.	0 98	Acc. contains b
3.	1 97	,, ,, $b - c$
4.	3 00	,, ,, $10b - 10c$
5.	1 98	,, ,, $9b - 10c$
6.	0 97	,, ,, $9b - 9c$
7.	0 99	,, ,, $a + 9b - 9c$
8.	6 00	Output $a+9b-9c$
9.	7 00	Stop

be used instead. Some indication of what is involved is described later in this chapter.

So far, we have assumed that the data a, b and c is actually in the storage registers 99, 98 and 97, and we must now consider how this is achieved. First, the three numbers a, b and c are punched on, say, paper-tape, which is, in turn, presented to the input channel of the computer (Figure 9) which we assume is capable of 'reading' one number at a time. The program of instructions is as shown in the first eighteen storage registers of Figure 9, and when the start-button is pressed the control unit, as already described, takes the first instruction 5 00, decodes it, and closes the corresponding switch. Closing the switch 5 has the effect of transferring the number a from the input register to the accumulator, *as well as* automatically advancing the data-tape through the input mechanism to read b; thus, as a result of this first instruction, the accumulator contains a, and the input register contains b; the second instruction 4 99 closes switches 4 and 99, and causes the contents of the accumulator to be written into register 99, leaving zero in the accumulator; the third instruction 5 00, transfers the number b from the input register to the accumulator, while the input channel automatically advances the data-tape to read c; thus, the accumulator contains b and the input register contains c; the fourth instruction transfers the accumulator contents to register 98, which thus contains b, while the accumulator now contains zero; the fifth instruction 5 00 transfers c from the input register to the accumulator, while the input channel advances the data-tape to read nothing since all numbers have now been read; the sixth instruction 4 97 writes the accumulator contents to register 97, leaving the accumulator empty; the rest of the instructions are identical with those described earlier for obtaining $11a + 12b + c$.

It is in this way that, on pressing the start button, the computer mechanism automatically carries out one instruction at a time, and so reads in the data, performs the calculation, and finally ejects the result via the output register to a teleprinter (or a tape-punch, or other output device), and stops. The data is actually read in by the program. (To the inevitable question as to how the program itself gets into the computer, suffice it to say that it gets in by means of a special program—often called the initial orders—always kept in the computer, and supplied by the manufacturer when the machine is delivered from the factory.)

The elementary computer operations 0, 1, 2, 3, 4, 5, 6, 7, which the control unit can decode and execute, are called the *order code* of the computer. There is no reason, of course, other than economic, why any computer should be confined to this limited set of basic operations—

0	add
1	subtract
2	clear
3	left shift
4	write
5	input
6	output
7	stop

and in practice one often finds others: multiply, divide, collate. There are only about a dozen essentially different types in all, since more complex functions, used less frequently, can be programmed.

It will be noticed that all the basic operations in the order code (except the 'stop' instruction) involve some elementary transaction with the accumulator. To relieve pressure on this bottleneck it is common practice to have not one accumulator but several, and for this reason the order code must be appropriately extended, so that, for example 21 means 'clear accumulator one' and 24 means 'clear accumulator four'. Similarly, a computer will need one input register associated with input device, and one output register associated with each output device; hence, the order code may get further complicated, 253 for example, meaning 'input from input register 2 to accumulator 3'. No new principle is involved, however, it is merely the extension of the order code to cope with multiple facilities.

IMPORTANT PROGRAMMING TECHNIQUES

So far so good, but few calculations or procedures proceed quite so simply. Usually, choices between courses of action have to be made. For example, even in a simple tax calculation one must decide whether or not the residual income exceeds or does not exceed a certain amount so that taxed rates are charged accordingly, and this will obviously influence the course of the calculation in a particular case. In compiling statistics from medical records a human clerk must decide whether or not a patient is in a certain age group, of a certain sex, in a specified disease category, and so on. Even in these cases, and certainly in all cases for which a computer is used, the calculation or procedure does not proceed in one direct sequence, instruction by instruction from the first to the last, but must 'branch' from one course of action to another as the problem demands. Therefore, if any one of these tasks is to be automated, some 'decision' technique must be evolved for dealing with it.

The astonishing thing is, as the great computer pioneer Charles Babbage recognised over 100 years ago, all decisions can be broken down by analysis into discriminating between either positive and negative or zero and non-zero. The following elementary example illustrates the technique, rather than the power, of the method. Suppose we require the computer automatically to 'read' in two numbers a and b, 'decide' which is the largest, and print out the answer. The computer will need to subtract b from a and, depending on whether the result is positive or negative, choose a or b accordingly. This can be accomplished by the program shown overleaf.

The first four instructions of the program 'input' a and b into registers 99 and 98, and the next two instructions form $a - b$ in the accumulator. However, at this point the program 'branches' and must somehow be made to follow instructions 8, 9, 10 if the accumulator is positive, and instructions 11, 12, 13, 14 if the accumulator is negative. Instructions 8, 9, 10 simply change

126 *Medical Automation*

Program   *Explanation*
1. 5 00 read in *a* from input register ⎫ these four instructions
2. 4 99 write *a* to register 99   ⎪ effectively input *a* and
3. 5 00 read in *b* from input register ⎬ *b* into registers
4. 4 98 write *b* to register 98   ⎭ 99 & 98.

5. 0 99 add *a* into accumulator   ⎫ these two instructions
6. 1 98 subtract *b* from accumulator   ⎬ form *a-b* in accumu-
                                          ⎭ lator

   positive   │   negative

 8. 0 98   11. 2 00
 9. 6 00   12. 0 98
10. 7 00   13. 6 00
                     14. 7 00

a — *b* into *a*, transfer *a* to the output register and stop, while instructions 11, 12, 13, 14 clear the accumulator; insert *b* into the accumulator, transfer *b* to the output register and stop. The problem, of course, is how to effect the branching automatically. This is achieved by writing the program as follows—

```
         1.   5  00
         2.   4  99
         3.   5  00
         4.   4  98
         5.   0  99
         6.   1  98
    ┌────7.   8  11    branching instruction
    │    8.   0  98
    │    9.   6  00
    │   10.   7  00
    └──→11.   2  00
        12.   0  98
        13.   6  00
        14.   7  00
```

All instructions are exactly as before except for the seventh instruction, called the '*branching instruction*'. This involves a new operation given code number 8. The control unit, in the usual way, takes each instruction in turn, decodes it and closes the appropriate switches, but when it reaches the branching instruction, 8 11, it inspects the sign of the accumulator; if this is positive it does nothing and simply carries on to the next instruction, but if it is negative it 'jumps' to instruction 11 as specified in the address-part of the branching instruction. By this simple but ingenious convention a program can be caused to follow one course of action rather than another according to some pre-set criteria. Just as this number 8 instruction jumps the sequence, or carries on the sequence, according to whether the accumulator is negative or positive, so another instruction, say number 9, is usually available which jumps the sequence, or carries on the sequence, according to whether the accumulator is zero or not zero. This is particularly useful if one is trying to identify characteristics. For example, if one is searching records (the storage of alphabetical data is dealt with shortly) to ascertain how many males there are, one simply 'subtracts' the word male from the word male or female, as the case may be, on each record. Males minus male gives a zero result, whereas female minus male is not zero (whatever else it is!). Similarly, to find additionally the number of males with measles, one simply 'subtracts' measles from the disease item on each record, knowing that this will yield zero only in the case of patients with measles. And so on.

In the simple example given above there is only one branching function; in more complex examples the branching network may be quite intricate, offering a variety of courses of action that depend on multiple criteria being satisfied. Although in each and every case one might say that a computer is 'deciding what to do', it is evident that the *strategy* of choice is fully determined by the program designer, even though what choice is actually made in a particular case depends upon the data supplied.

Another feature of all the examples used so far, which is atypical, is that each instruction is obeyed only once. Since a machine can obey as many as a million instructions a second, a program in which each instruction was obeyed only once, and that lasted for an hour, would consist of 3,600 million instructions. Understandably therefore, an essential feature of program writing, in fact much of the art and technique of it, is in devising minimum sequences of instructions that can be *repeated* many times. This is most commonly accomplished by using a branching instruction n the framework of a 'loop organisation', and what this means is illustrated by the following arrangement for performing a particular task 1,000 times.

Loop Organisation

1. Store the number—1000 (called a 'count') in a register.
2. Perform the task (specified by a suitable program) once.
3. Add 1 to the count.
4. If count negative jump back to step 2; if positive proceed.
5. Stop.

From this it can be seen that a program for performing a particular task many times has to be written only once; it is then incorporated in steps 1, 3 and 4, above, in order to perform it 1,000 times. After the task has been performed exactly 1,000 times the procedure will come to an end. Step 4, which in effect 'decides' whether the count is complete or not, is achieved by using the branching instruction number 8. Also, by changing the 'count' number to any other number, the number of times the task is repeated is changed accordingly.

An even more powerful technique in program design is that whereby a program is made to *modify itself automatically so as to alter its action as it proceeds*. This is possible since a program acts by operating on stored data; in particular, therefore, it can be arranged to act on those numbers which form its own instructions, thereby changing the instructions and therefore itself, too, as it proceeds. This is especially useful in repetitive tasks; for example, there is no point in performing a tax calculation on the same salary 1,000 times; there is no point in selecting data from the same medical record 1,000 times; the program must in these cases modify its action on each successive cycle to enable it to act on a different salary or a different medical record. More ambitious applications of this technique enable programs to adapt themselves, or improve themselves, in a manner similar to human learning. A fairly typical example of this kind of thing is the chess-playing procedure briefly described in chapter One. There we indicated that in deciding which move to select against a particular player, the programmed procedure should weight its choice according to the relative success of these moves as recorded from previous games; in other words its action should be modified by weighting factors that will change from game to game. Similar considerations would apply to computer-assisted diagnosis in which relative specificities (used as weighting factors in determining final probabilities) were updated frequently from new clinical statistics. And, because a computer never tires, because it can on every decision-making occasion exhaust all alternatives, and because it can 'memorise' (store) quantitatively all that has gone before—which human decision-makers cannot do—it is possible for the computer procedure to exceed the performance of its designer.

This stresses a very important point. It is often said, and rightly, that a computer's actions are limited to what it can be ordered to perform; but how limited is that? If a strategy of improvement can be explicitly formulated, it is by no means inconceivable that the improvement may go well beyond the extent to which the unaided cerebral faculties can take it at 'handraulic' speeds. No new principles are *called for, therefore, other than the methods already described, to explain how a computer procedure may exceed the performance of its designer.*

HIGH-LEVEL LANGUAGES

The reader, now mindful of the tedious detail involved in formulating detailed machine code programs for even the simplest of calculations, will wonder how on earth it is ever possible to design programs for more complex procedures. The key lies in what are called 'sub-routines', short sequences of instructions, i.e. short programs, which once designed and tested can be used again and again, and subsequent users need not know in detail how they are constructed. All they need to know is that this particular sub-routine takes the square root of a number, that another sorts numbers into order, that another tabulates this variable against that, and so on; code names such as SQRT, SORT and TABULATE are used to identify the sub-routines. When a particular type of computer has been in operation for some time, there will exist many hundreds of useful sub-routines, constituting what is generally called a 'library of sub-routines'. The value of this library in terms of the investment involved will invariably exceed the cost of the computer itself. It represents the 'software' as it is generally called, without which the physical 'hardware'—the mechanism described earlier—would be useless.

The existence of a library of sub-routines considerably influences the way in which large programming problems are tackled, the object being to break them down into sub-programs chosen as far as possible to fit existing sub-routines, so that only residual sub-programs have to be developed from scratch.

An even more important development, which is a main feature of present day practice, is what might be called the 'purpose-built' library of sub-routines. Essentially this consists of using professional programmers to create a repertoire of many hundreds of basic sub-routines, designed with the objective of enabling any particular program to be made up by combining the basic sub-routines in some particular order. This is analogous to basic English, which is an attempt to create a minimal vocabulary that will enable any particular sentence or message to be formulated entirely from the basic English vocabulary. The analogy goes further since each of the basic sub-routines in the purpose-built library is given a code name such as PRINT, READ, SUM, SORT, SQRT, and so on. A particular program can then be compiled by using *only these code names* in some particular sequence.

The entire set of code names constitutes a vocabulary, and it, plus the rules or syntax (or grammar) by which the words in the vocabulary can be combined, is called a *computer language*, or more frequently a *high-level* language, since it enables a programmer to use words or phrases which resemble ordinary, everyday language. COBOL, FORTRAN, and ALGOL are three of the most widely used computer languages. COBOL (COmmercial and Business Oriented Language) is used principally for business data-processing where the processing of files of records is a principal feature; FORTRAN (FORmula TRANslator) and ALGOL (ALGebraic Oriented Language) are most frequently used for computational procedures. By the use of such high-level languages the programmer is substantially relieved of the detailed machine-code programming described earlier in this chapter.

However, the very nature of a computer mechanism is such, as we have learned, that it can execute a program only in machine-code form, and it should be emphasised that the use of a high-level language by the programmer thereby places an additional task on the computer, namely translating from high-level language form into machine code form. This is achieved by means of a substantial program called a Compiler, Assembler, or Autocode. Basically, each of these consists of a purpose-built library of sub-routines, a dictionary of their code names and a translator routine. Under the control of the translator routine, each word or phrase ('statement') of the high-level language is read into the computer. It is compared with each word or phrase in the dictionary to ascertain its identity (a massive understatement of what happens in detail), and then the particular sub-routine(s) to which it refers is extracted. In this way the machine-code version of the high-level program is systematically compiled (hence, Compiler), or assembled (hence, Assembler), or automatically coded (hence, Autocode).

No computer manufacturer today supplies a computer without one (or more) of these compilers, which represents a substantial investment on his part since the development of each usually requires many tens of programmer years. For the user it means that he can begin to use a computer without knowing how it works in detail. All he has to do is to learn the conventions of a high-level computer language, which, depending on aptitude, may be of the order of a week or so—comparable with the effort required to learn to drive a motor-car—followed by plenty of practice. In fact, following the driving analogy, the user of a high-level language is rather like the driver of a car with an automatic gear box: neither needs to know the details of changing down or up as it is attended to automatically.

It would be wrong to give the impression that high-level languages have entirely displaced machine-code programming, although the trend is that way. The great variety of possible applications of computers has prevented the realisation of a truly universal computer language that could be used for all purposes and be accepted by all makes of computer, although the search continues. Particular languages have particular merits in particular areas of application, and for this reason computer languages continue to be invented. As computer application in medicine extends, someone somewhere is sure to propose the merits of a special computer language, say MEDOL (MEDically Oriented Language), but until that time should arrive, if it ever does, COBOL, FORTRAN and ALGOL are likely to meet many of the requirements, with occasional excursions into machine code, where its advantages outweigh the tedium involved. We should not rule out the possibility of a special language being developed for communication via data-terminals in real-time applications.

Meanwhile, the simple advice to a newcomer is 'learn a computer language'; when one has been learnt, it is a relatively simpler task to learn another.

BINARY: AN ENGINEERING EXPEDIENT

The whole of the exposition throughout this book has thus far managed to avoid any discussion of binary, and with it the risk of inducing the well-known syndrome of 'binary trauma'. This is as it should be because the overwhelming justification for binary is its simplification of the engineering problems; just how, we hope to show now. The design of every practical digital computer is dominated by the needs:

(a) to store alphabetical and numerical data reliably and cheaply;

(b) to operate on the data at very high speeds

Clearly, there would be considerable practical advantages in retaining the 26-letter (A to Z), and 10-digit (0 to 9) alphabets in the engineering solution, but, as we shall see, the economic disadvantages are so great, that this is hardly ever done except for special purposes. This does not matter very much as the number of symbols in an alphabet has no bearing on what can be articulated in terms of that alphabet; in fact, any message or statement written in terms of the familiar alphabets of 26 symbols, and 10 symbols, can just as readily be re-stated in an alphabet of 1 symbol, or 2 symbols, or 3 symbols, and so on. In choosing the most convenient alphabet for engineering computers, therefore, any number of symbols can be chosen.

Consider an alphabet of only one symbol denoted, say, by the letter O. The number of words that can be formed consisting of only one symbol in this alphabet is obviously one, namely the word O; the number of words consisting of two symbols is also one, namely OO; the number of words consisting of three symbols is also one, namely the word OOO; in fact, the number of words consisting of x symbols is also one, namely the word formed from x Os. But, it will be noticed, there is no limit to the number of words that can be formed; a vocabulary of 8,000 words or even 18,000 words could certainly be represented by using an alphabet of only one symbol. It would, of course, not be a very convenient language, and for this reason it need not be pursued further.

The next simplest alphabet to consider is that consisting of two symbols, which we will denote by 0 and 1. The number of words consisting of just one symbol in this 'binary' alphabet is clearly two, namely 0 and 1; the number of words consisting of two symbols is evidently four because each of the one-letter words can be associated with both 0 and 1, yielding—

$$00$$
$$01$$
$$10$$
$$11$$

By associating an 0-symbol with each of these four two-letter words, and also a 1-symbol with each of them, it can be seen that the number of three-letter words is eight, namely

$$000$$
$$001$$
$$010$$
$$011$$
$$100$$
$$101$$
$$110$$
$$111$$

By associating an 0-symbol with each of these eight three-letter words, and a 1-symbol with each of them, it can be seen that the number of four-letter words is sixteen, and so on. In fact, the number of one-letter words is 2, the number of two-letter words is 2×2 (2^2), the number of three-letter words is $2 \times 2 \times 2$ (2^3), the number of four-letter words $2 \times 2 \times 2 \times 2$ (2^4), and so on, as shown by the following table—

$$2^1 = 2$$
$$2^2 = 4$$
$$2^3 = 8$$
$$2^4 = 16$$
$$2^5 = 32$$
$$2^6 = 64$$
$$2^7 = 128$$
$$2^8 = 256$$
$$2^9 = 512$$
$$2^{10} = 1,024$$
$$2^{11} = 2,048$$
$$2^{12} = 4,096$$
$$2^{13} = 8,192$$
$$2^{14} = 16,384 \text{ and so on}$$

Thus, there is no limit to the number of words that can be formed, and moreover a vocabulary of, say, 8,000 words could be represented by 8,000 binary words of no more than thirteen symbols each, which is quite reasonable. Because of this fact, because of its simplicity, and for reasons of eminent practicality in terms of electronic devices, the binary language is the one most commonly (almost universally) used in modern computer design, and, after a short digression, we shall consider its application in greater detail.

Before doing so, however, consider the alphabet of 26 symbols denoted in the usual way by A, B, C, . . ., Z. The number of words of one letter that can be formed is obviously 26; by associating A with all 26, B with all 26, C with all 26, and so on, it can be seen that the number of two-letter words that can be formed is $26 \times 26 = 676$; by associating A with all 676, B with all 676, and so on, the number of three-letter words that can be formed is $26 \times 26 \times 26 = 17,576$; the number of four-letter words is $26 \times 26 \times 26 \times 26 = 26^4$, and so on. In fact, the number of seven-letter words that can be formed from 26 letters exceeds 8,000,000,000, a fact worth pondering when we consider that most people's vocabularies stop far short of 8,000 words. It means that if a computer were engineered on the basis of a 26-letter alphabet, purely for the practical convenience of preserving the familiar alphabet, then much less than one-millionth of its information capacity would be utilised. That in a nutshell is why it is not used. Perhaps the principal advantages of the 26-letter alphabet are euphony (not always in evidence) and redundancy, by which we mean that so many word arrangements are not used that two different people can badly mis-spell 'pneumonia', and still a third person would be able to recognise what he was trying to spell. An electronic digital computer which ingests data silently has no need of euphony, and can find more effective ways of using the advantages of redundancy without having to be over-engineered a million-fold.

To return now to the binary alphabet. Ordinary words and numbers can be translated into binary in a variety of ways of varying merits. We shall first describe one of the two most common representations used which assigns a binary code to each letter or digit. Since there are 26 letters and 10 numerical digits, a minimum of 36 symbols must be represented. A five-letter

Computers: Physical Attributes

Letter	6-bit Binary Code	5-Hole Tape	Misc. Symbols and Figures	6-bit Binary Code	5-Hole Tape
A	100001	••••o	1	000001	••••o
B	100010	•••o•	2	000010	•••o•
C	100011	•••oo	*	000011	•••oo
D	100100	••o••	4	000100	••o••
E	100101	••o•o	$	000101	••o•o
F	100110	••oo•	=	000110	••oo•
G	100111	••ooo	7	000111	••ooo
H	101000	•o•••	8	001000	•o•••
I	101001	•o••o	,	001001	•o••o
J	101010	•o•o•	,	001010	•o•o•
K	101011	•o•oo	+	001011	•o•oo
L	101100	•oo••	:	001100	•oo••
M	101101	•oo•o	—	001101	•oo•o
N	101110	•ooo•	.	001110	•ooo•
O	101111	•oooo	%	001111	•oooo
P	110000	o••••	o	010000	o••••
Q	110001	o•••o	(	010001	o•••o
R	110010	o••o•	)	010010	o••o•
S	110011	o••oo	3	010011	o••oo
T	110100	o•o••	?	010100	o•o••
U	110101	o•o•o	5	010101	o•o•o
V	110110	o•oo•	6	010110	o•oo•
W	110111	o•ooo	/	010111	o•ooo
X	111000	oo•••	8	011000	oo•••
Y	111001	oo••o	9	011001	oo••o
Z	111010	oo•o•	£	011010	oo•o•
Figure Shift	111011	oo•oo	Figure Shift	011011	oo•oo
Space	111100	ooo••	Space	011100	ooo••
Carriage Return	111101	ooo•o	Carriage Return	011101	ooo•o
Line Feed	111110	oooo•	Line Feed	011110	oooo•
Letter Shift	111111	ooooo	Letter Shift	011111	ooooo

Figure 10. Six-bit representation of alpha-numeric characters

binary code cannot be used since there are only $2^5 = 32$ five-letter binary codes. We must, therefore, use a six-letter binary code of which there are $2^6 = 64$ in all. These can be assigned in any way and Figure 10 shows a typical representation used in practice. The second column from the left shows the 6-bit* codes repre-

*'Bit' is a commonly used abbreviation for binary digit.

senting each letter, and the second column from the right shows the 6-bit codes representing each decimal digit. The significance of the '5-hole tape' columns will be explained later. Since only 36 codes are used for letters and digits, the remaining 28 are used for other purposes, which need not concern us except to note that every code is used and none is wasted. Each of the 64 symbols is generally called a *character*. The numerical digits are not set out consecutively because they are arranged to have an odd number of 1s in their codes, this feature being used by the computer for automatic error detection. All the letter codes have a 1 at the beginning of their 6-bit codes, while all the decimal digits have a 0 at the beginning of theirs. The main point to note about this table is that once a 6-bit code is used *the familiar distinction between letters and numbers disappears*. It is not so fundamental a distinction as habit might lead us to think, and *a computer can therefore process both with equal facility in a common alphabet*; indeed, as the table indicates, 28 other miscellaneous symbols (not letters of decimal digits) can also be treated in a similar way. This is why a computer is not basically a calculator. Only if the 6-bit symbols represent the digits 0 to 9, and the program embodies rules of calculation, will the computer be acting as a calculator. If, however, the symbols represent chess-pieces and a program embodies rules of play, then the computer will be able to 'play' chess—as described in chapter One.

Physical Attributes

It should now be evident that any word, phrase or number can easily be translated into binary by assigning to each letter or digit its appropriate 6-bit code. One of the commonest ways of achieving this physically is by means of key-board punching: given a key-board arrangement similar to a typewriter, with as many keys as there are codes in the table above, and such that when a key is pressed it not only types out a symbol in the familiar style, but also punches out the corresponding code on paper tape, when the 6-bit codes are generated physically—holes and not-holes respectively representing 1s and 0s. As a matter of history, 5-hole teletape, used in telecommunications, was quickly adapted to computer use, and is still used either for reasons of expediency (the investment has been made), or advantage (compatible transmission facilities). Its ambiguity, however, when used for alpha-numeric representation has to be faced (Figure 11). The main problem is that the leading bit distinguishing letters from digits is missing, so that, for example, BABY is indistinguishable from 2129 (Figure 11). This is usually solved by preceding letters with a 'letter-shift' code, and numbers by a 'figure-shift' code, by pressing the letter-shift key on the keyboard before typing on letters, and pressing the figure-shift key before typing out numbers. When a 5-hole punched-paper tape prepared in this way is inserted into a computer, a suitably designed input programme can, by detecting the letter-shift and figure-shift codes, augment the ensuing 5-hole codes with the appropriate leading bit. Tapes with other numbers of holes are also used in practice, and similar considerations apply, but since we are only concerned here to give some appreciation of the principal physical attributes of computers these will not be discussed.

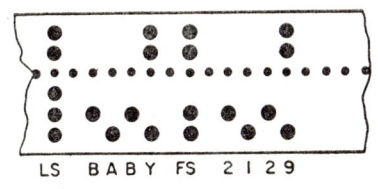

Figure 11. Distinguishing letters from numbers on five-hole tape

Having considered how both data and program, by means of keyboard punching, can be represented physically in 6-bit binary form, the next stage is to consider how these 6-bit codes are physically dealt with inside the computer. Two-state devices, capable of representing binary codes, are readily available to electronic engineers in the form of diodes, transistors (suitably coupled), and magnetic fields. The latter is most commonly used to make up the storage registers of the central processor. Most readers are familiar with the properties of magnets (ferrite material). A simple bar magnet can be magnetised in one of two directions (a two-state device). It can be quickly switched from one state of magnetisation to another by wrapping it round with a coil of wire and passing an electric current through the wire one way or the other (electrically switchable at upwards of a million times a second); moreover, by bending the bar magnet round into the shape of a core it will retain its state of magnetisation for long periods (stable). Here, then, is an ideal device for storing a binary digit: *a ferrite core* (Plate 8B). A storage register made up of say, 36 ferrite cores (each a millimetre or so in diameter) will store half-a-dozen 6-bit symbols. A typical 'ferrite core store' module will comprise 64×64 ($= 4{,}096$) 36-bit registers; and a central processor will usually contain a number of such modules, thereby having a capacity of many thousands of ferrite core registers. Since a register (in this case) can hold six characters, and since a character may be a digit or a letter, registers are commonly called 'words'. Also, the number $2^{10} = 1{,}024$ occurs so frequently in binary (as does the number 1,000 in decimal working) that it is usually denoted by the letter K. Hence, a typical phrase: 'the central processor has a ferrite core store containing 32K words of storage'—a perfectly reasonable piece of jargon once you know what it means.

Ferrite cores are predominantly used to make up the fast active store of the central processor in almost all computer systems. They have established their supremacy for over a decade over many other physical devices with which they once competed, and the prospect is that they will continue to provide this function well into the 1970s although they are being replaced gradually by cheaper, less bulky semiconductor stores. Ferrite cores can be used to make up storage registers of different lengths, which are usually chosen to be a multiple number of characters. Since characters on punched tape, for example, are input one character at a time, they can, under the control of a suitable input program, be 'packed' into the ferrite core storage registers. If, for instance, a medical record contains some 720 characters that have been transferred to punched paper-tape, and thence transferred to a ferrite core store comprising 6-character storage registers, then the medical record data will occupy $720 \div 6 = 120$ storage registers.

Because the accumulator registers, and the elementary computer operations (discussed earlier in this chapter) are used relatively more frequently (one or other of them being involved with every program instruction) than the ferrite core registers, then faster computer speeds can be achieved by making these devices up from faster switching components than ferrite cores. Transistors, which can be switched a hundred or more times faster than ferrite cores, are widely used for this purpose. In fact, their switching times are measured not in millionths of a second, but in what are called nano-seconds (a nano-second is one-thousandth part of a millionth of a second). This is the common time domain for most computer engineers these days, although at the research end an increasing amount of work is done in pico-seconds, a pico-second being one-millionth part of a millionth of a second. Since electricity travels about a foot in one nano-second. the length of wire joining components would have been a serious problem were it not for the advent of micro-miniaturisation, which reduces the sizes and distances between components to microscopic dimensions.

To summarise then: information in character-units is transferred by means of input devices to multiple-character ferrite core registers. Under program control, these characters can be transferred between the ferrite core registers and the accumulators via one or other of the elementary computer operations, and be 'processed' accordingly. Finally, character units can be transferred via an output register and 'filed' on bulk magnetic stores (tapes, discs, drums), and when wanted transferred back via an input register to the ferrite core store for processing. A computer, therefore, is basically a binary, or character, shunting engine, capable of performing only the most elementary operations, but able because of its phenomenal speed to do enough of these elementary operations a second to execute data-procedures of astonishing complexity. It is programming that bridges the gap between the two, and that analyses a useful data-procedure into a detailed prescription of elementary operations. Fortunately, this tedious travail is increasingly facilitated by high-level languages of one sort or another.

Appendix 2
Natural Binary

Although the 6-bit alpha-numeric representation, which involves assigning a 6-bit code to each letter and digit to convert it to binary form, has the virtue of simplicity for didactic purposes, and is in fact one of the two most common representations used, it has conspicuous disadvantages in certain situations of which the reader should be made aware.

The first type of disadvantage is lack of economy. This is apparent from the fact that if the word 'carcinoma', for example, were represented by nine 6-bit characters, then 54 bits would be required in all, enough in fact to distinguish any one of 16,000,000,000,000,000 words. Obviously this is greatly in excess of what is required. If, in using the word 'carcinoma', a doctor really only wished to differentiate between, say, one of 1,000 categories, then a 10-bit representation ($2^{10} = 1,024$) of 'carcinoma' would be adequate. Similarly, it is very inefficient to use a 6-bit coded character (M or F) to denote sex, since 6 bits enables some 64 ($2^6 = 64$) different possibilities to be distinguished and only two are wanted in most situations; one bit is sufficient. Even any 3-digit number (000 to 999), which requires 18 bits when three 6-bit characters are used, can be represented by 10 bits. One therefore needs to be on guard in thinking purely in terms of characters (which people whose experience has been largely in the milieu of punched-card data-processing equipment have a marked tendency to do), otherwise four-fifths or more of computer capacity will be wasted, a fact of which many organisations are only slowly becoming aware. The important thing is not characters, but the 'information content' of a word or phrase (which can be elicited by enumerating and assigning the frequency of each word or phrase category) in order to establish an efficient binary representation. Strictly, this is the province of operational research, and unless computer data-procedures are subjected to this kind of analysis at the very start, then almost certainly computers will be used (are used) with a degree of inefficiency that only ignorance could possibly tolerate.

The second type of disadvantage of the 6-bit alpha-numeric representation is that it does not conform directly with the rules of arithmetic and, therefore, is not generally used for computational work.

Both these disadvantages are overcome by using the 'natural binary representation', so-called because it does obey the laws of the natural numbers 1, 2, 3, 4 ... and so on. (This representation and 6-bit alpha-numeric representation are the two most commonly used in practice.) For example, consider the number 109, whose binary equivalent is 1101101. Just as each digit in 109 indicates an ascending power of 10, so each bit in 1101101 indicates an ascending power of 2, and this feature indicates how to convert any decimal number into its natural binary

10^2	10	1	2^6	2^5	2^4	2^3	2^2	2	1
1	0	9	1	1	0	1	1	0	1

equivalent, namely, by successively dividing by 2, thus—

2)	109		
2)	54	remainder	1
2)	27	,,	0
2)	13	,,	1
2)	6	,,	1
2)	3	,,	0
2)	1	,,	1
2)	0	,,	1

Thus, 1101101 is the natural binary equivalent of 109. Another systematic feature of natural numbers is that by adding unity, one produces the next number in sequence; this is also true of natural binary, thus—

```
   109              1101101
     1                    1
   ___              _____
   110              1101110
```

Adding 1 to 9 in decimals results in '0 and carry 1'; equally, adding 1 to 1 in binary results in '0 and carry 1'. If the reader finds this strange and novel he should remember (if he is British) that he has in fact been doing it all his life when he adds up the ten shillings column of his accounts: 1 (10/-) plus 1 (10/-) equals '0 and carry 1'.

In applying the natural binary representation to alphabetical data one starts with a dictionary (or list) of, say, 1,000 words and assigns to each word, in turn, a natural binary 10-bit number; e.g. the 109th word in the list is represented by 0001101101, which is, as we have already remarked, considerably less than the 54-bit representation that would result from a 6-bit alphanumeric representation. One point: it is important to note that *the user does not* (unless he wishes) *have to deal directly in binary*, but only the programmer; it is he who must decide on the most efficient representation for a particular purpose, and must strike a reasonable balance between the considerations referred to.

Glossary of Technical Terms

The major source is the glossary in the C.S.D. Management Studies Report No. 2, 'Computers in Central Government Ten Years Ahead' (1971).

Terms in common use and explained in this book are not generally included.

ACCESS TIME	Of a computer store. The time interval between the instant the control unit calls for a transfer of data to or from the store and the instant this operation is completed.
ACOUSTIC MEMORY	A term applied to storage devices which exploit, by their design, the properties of sound transmission through various materials.
ALGOL	ALGOrithmic language: A process-oriented language developed as a result of internal co-operation to develop a standard language for expressing computational algorithms.
ANALOGUE	Pertaining to data represented in the form of continuously variable physical quantities (e.g. voltage or angular position). Contrast with digital.
APPLICATION	The problem or system to which a computer (or other processing equipment or technique) is applied.
APPLICATION PACKAGE	A computer routine or set of routines designed for a specific application (e.g.

inventory control, on-line savings accounting, linear programming, etc.)

Note: In most cases, the routines in the application packages are necessarily written in a generalised way and will need to be modified to meet each user's own specific needs.

ARCHITECTURE
A term loosely applied to the basic design of computers embracing, *inter alia*, the word length, instruction code, and the interrelationship between the main parts of the computer.

BACKING STORE
A store of much larger capacity than the working store, but of longer access time. Data may be transferred in blocks.

BATCH PROCESSING
A technique in which items to be processed are collected into groups (i.e. 'batched') to permit convenient and efficient processing.

Note: Most business applications are of the batch processing type; the records of all transactions affecting a particular master file are accumulated over a period of time (e.g. one day), then they are arranged in sequence and processed against the master file.

BENCH-MARK
A precisely defined problem that is coded and timed for a number of computers in order to measure their performance in a meaningful and directly comparable manner.

BUREAU
A general term for a computer installation available for processing data on behalf of many users. The range of services undertaken by the bureau (e.g. systems design, programming) will vary according to the needs of the users and from bureau to bureau. Bureaux will also vary in the degree to which they are dedicated to given tasks.

Glossary

BYTE	A group of adjacent bits operated upon as a unit and usually shorter than a word.

Note: In a number of important current computer systems, the term 'byte' has been assigned the more specific meaning of a group of eight adjacent bits which can represent one alphanumeric character or two decimal digits. |
CAD	*See* Computer-aided Design.
CENTRAL PROCESSOR	The central processor is that part of an automatic data processing system that is not considered as peripheral equipment.
CHARACTER	A member of a set of agreed elements, intended for use in conveying information either when arranged together in an agreed fashion (in general sequentially) or when isolated. Each member has one or more conventional representations on paper and in equipment. The most common characters are the letters of the alphabet and the ten arabic numerals.
COBOL	Common Business Orientated Language. A process-orientated language developed to facilitate the preparation and interchange of programs to perform business data processing functions.
CODE	An agreed set of unambiguous rules used to specify the way in which data may be represented by the characters of a character set.
COMPATIBILITY	The characteristic that enables one device to accept and process data prepared by another device without prior code translation, data transcription or other modifications. Thus, one computer system is 'data compatible' with another if it can read and process the punched cards, magnetic tape, etc, produced by the other computer.

COMPILER — A program designed to transform (e.g. translate, assemble and structure) orograms expressed in terms of one language (e.g. a procedure orientated language) into equivalent programs expressed in terms of a computer language or a language of similar form. A compiling program may often include an assembly program, a generating program, and a diagnostic program.

COMPUTER-AIDED DESIGN — The use of a computer as part of a design task, e.g. for steel structures, electronic circuits.

COMPUTER SERIES — Especially in recent years, manufacturers have introduced ranges of computers with similar architecture. Each range is known as a series. Within each series there may be differences in processing speed, size of stores, number of peripherals, size of instruction code, etc. A considerable degree of compatibility exists between the computers within a series.

CONFIGURATION — A specific set of equipment units that are interconnected and (in the case of a computer) pro-configuration consists of one or more central processors, one or more storage devices, and one or more input-output devices.

CONSOLE — In automatic data processing an assembly of displays, manual controls etc. for use by the operator or engineer of a computer.

CONVERSATIONAL MODE — A mode of operation that implies a 'dialogue' between a computer and its user, in which the computer program examines the input supplied by the user and formulates questions or comments which are directed back to the user.

CORAL — Computer Orientated Real-time Applications language.

Glossary 147

CORE STORAGE — A type of storage that uses an array of magnetic cores, each capable of storing one bit of data.

Note: Most current computers use magnetic core storage as their main working storage. This widespread acceptance is due to the fact that magnetic cores require no power while storing data, can be switched rapidly from one state to the other by relatively small currents, and can tolerate adverse environmental conditions.

DATA BANK — A representation of facts for a large collection of data of similar kind, usually in coded form and usually amassed gradually. The data in a bank is normally organised to be usable for multiple purposes. Generally synonymous with Data Base.

DATA BASE — *See* Data Bank.

DATA CONCENTRATOR — A term used in data transmission to denote an electronic device for receiving data (usually at slow speed from several sources), organising and storing it, and subsequently transmitting it (usually at higher speed to a computer). The converse happens with outgoing transmission.

DATA LINK — The means by which (e.g. telephone line, microwave) data transmission takes place.

DATA TRANSMISSION — The transmission between remote points of data in coded form by means of signals (usually electrical).

DEDICATION — A loose term used to describe the extent to which a computer installation is confined to some given task or group of allied tasks.

DIGIT — A single character that represents an integer. That is in decimal notation, one of the characters 0 to 9.

DIRECT ACCESS — Pertaining to a storage device in which the access time is not significantly affected by the location of the data to be accessed; thus, any item of data that is stored on-line can be accessed within a relatively short time (usually less than one second).

DISC — A magnetic store in which the magnetic medium is on the surface of one or more rotating discs.

DRUM — A magnetic store in which the magnetic medium is on the curved surface of a rotating cylinder.

DUMP (TO) — To retain by storage elsewhere the contents of a set of locations either because the locations are temporarily required for another purpose or as a safeguard, e.g. against power failure, or for a check.

EMULATION — The process by which programs written for one computer may be run on a different computer. The conversation is carried out by hardware.

FILE — A collection of data, complete in some sense, for the purpose of a particular job. For example, in stock control a file could consist of the complete set of invoices for a given period. A file may be considered, where convenient, as composed of a number of records, each record containing the data relating to one particular part of a job. In the stock control example, each invoice could constitute one record.
A record may be further sub-divided into fields, each field being the smallest quantity of data considered as an entity for the purpose of the job. In the stock control example each line on an invoice could constitute a field.

FONT — A family or assortment of graphic character representations (i.e. a character set) of a particular size and style: e.g. Front E-13B, the MICR font adopted as a

	standard by the American Bankers' Association, and the USA Standard Optical Font for OCR.
FORMAT	The predetermined arrangement of data (e.g. characters, items, and lines), usually on a form or in a file.
FORTRAN	Formula Translating System: A process-orientated language designed to facilitate the preparation of computer programs to perform mathematical computations.
HARD COPY	Pertaining to documents containing data printed by data processing equipment in a form suitable for permanent retention (e.g. printed reports, listings, and logs).
HARDWARE	The apparatus, as opposed to the program or method of use. Readily detachable portions of the apparatus may be termed Equipment Units.
HIGHER LEVEL LANGUAGE	A language used for instructing the computer which is orientated to the problem to be resolved rather than to the operation of the computer. A program written in a higher level language is translated into machine language by a compiler. Examples: Algol, Cobol, Fortran, PLI.
HOUSEKEEPING	Pertaining to operations in a program or computer system which do not contribute directly to the solution of users' problems, but which are necessary in order to maintain control of the situation: e.g. the recording of the locations used by different parts of a program to ensure that data is not overwritten unless it is no longer required.
HYBRID COMPUTER	A combination of an analogue and a digital computer.
INFORMATION RETRIEVAL	The methods, procedures and equipment for recovering specific information from

stored data, especially from collections of documents or other graphic records.

INPUT — The process of transferring data from an external store or peripheral equipment to an internal store.

INTERACTIVE — Generally synonymous with 'conversational'.

INTERFACE — A shared boundary: e.g. the boundary between two systems, or between a computer and one of its peripheral devices.

INVERSE ADD TIME — The reciprocal of the time required to perform an addition. Usually expressed in mega-adds or kilo-adds per second.

LARGE SCALE INTEGRATION — A combination of many devices (transistor, diode and resistor) on a single integrated chip of silicon. An important development permitting much higher computing speeds.

LASER-HOLOGRAM — A type of storage making use of the minute interference patterns of light.

LSI — *See* Large Scale Integration.

MACHINE INSTRUCTION — An instruction that specifies a computer operation.

MACHINE LANGUAGE — A basic programming language consisting of machine instructions only.

MACHINE-READABLE FORM — Pertaining to data represented in a form that can be sensed by a data processing machine (e.g. by a card reader, magnetic tape unit, or optical character reader).

MAGNETIC INK CHARACTER RECOGNITION (MICR) — The automatic reading by machine of characters printed with magnetic ink.

MAGNETIC TAPE — A tape with a magnetic surface on which data can be stored by selective polarisation of portions of the surface.

Glossary 151

MAGNETO-OPTIC MEMORY
: A memory-utilising laser beam to change the direction of magnetism of a ferro-magnetic film.

MEMORY
: Same as store and storage.
A device intended for storage. The properties of a store depend upon the purposes for which it is intended: thus, a store forming part of an automatic data processing equipment may be controlled automatically, i.e. without human intervention.

MICR
: *See* Magnetic Ink Character Recognition.

MODULAR PROGRAMMING
: Methods of sub-dividing a program into smaller parts called modules. The advantages of modular programming include easier testing and better control of programming work. The rules governing the characteristics of such modules vary from method to method.

MULTI-ACCESS
: A generic term used to cover real-time, time-sharing, and remote batch-processing systems.

MULTI-PROCESSING
: The simultaneous execution of two or more sequences of instructions in a single computer system. This may be accomplished through the use of either two or more central processors (i.e. a multi-processor system) or a single central processor with several instruction registers and several sequence counters.

MULTI-PROGRAMMING
: A technique for handling simultaneously several programs related to various jobs by overlapping or interleaving their execution. The handling of the overlapping and interleaving execution of the various jobs is performed by a supervisory program; according to the priority requirements of the jobs it tries to optimise the performance of the system.

NUMERICAL CONTROL	The automatic control of operations (such as those of milling or boring machines) wherein the control is applied at discrete points in the operation through proper interpretation of numerical data.
OCR	*See* Optical Character Recognition.
ONE-SHOT	The execution of a number of different tasks in one computer process. For example, stores issue data may be used in one-shot to adjust outstanding stock balance, debit a cost account and, possibly, initiate re-ordering of stock.
ON-LINE	If one unit can be controlled by another without direct human intervention, the first unit is said to be on-line to the second. For example remote terminals are often connected on-line to a computer.
OPERATING SOFTWARE	A generic term to cover those general programs and routines necessary to the operation of a computer. Frequently provided by the computer manufacturer.
OPTICAL CHARACTER RECOGNITION	The automatic reading by machine of graphic characters through use of light-sensitive devices.
OUTPUT	The process of transferring data from an internal store to an external store or to peripheral equipment. The most frequent use applies to information provided in a readable form as the end-product of the computer process.
PACKAGE	*See* Application Package.
PACKING DENSITY	Of a data carrier, the number of storage cells per unit area or per unit length of track.
PAPER TAPE	A tape of defined dimensions designed to be punched with a pattern of holes in defined code positions for the purpose of recording data.

Glossary 153

PERIPHERAL EQUIPMENT (OR PERIPHERALS)	All of the input-output units and auxiliary storage units of a computer system.
PL1	A higher level language of wide scope intended to embrace both scientific and commercial applications. Largely developed by IBM, the only manufacturers who have yet issued PL1 compilers. Its future is controversial.
PROCESS	A system of operations designed to solve a problem or lead to a particular result.
(TO) READ	To obtain data from a store or data carrier. *Note*: In English usage, the use of the phrases 'to read to' and 'to write to' and 'to write from' by the viewpoint of the description. For example, the transfer of a block of data from a computer store to a peripheral store may be called 'writing to the peripheral store', or alternatively, 'reading from the computer store', or both.
READ-ONLY MEMORY	A memory containing permanent or quasi-permanent information used to facilitate the operation of the computer, to perform code conversion, etc.
REAL-TIME	Pertaining to a mode of operation in which the instants of concurrence of many events in the system satisfy restrictions determined by the occurrence of events in some other, independent system. For example, real-time operation is essential to computers associated with process control systems, message switching systems, and reservation systems.
REMOTE TERMINAL	An input or output device situated remotely from the computer but working to the computer by data link.
REPORT PROGRAM GENERATOR	A generator designed to construct programs to perform routine report-writing

154 Medical Automation

functions, e.g. to accept input data from punched cards or magnetic tape and produce printed reports, often with headings, sub-totals, etc.

RESPONSE TIME   The time-lag between the initiation of an input and delivery of the corresponding output.

SEARCH LANGUAGE   A higher level language specially designed to facilitate the retrieval of information from a computer file (data bank).

SERIES   *See* Computer Series.

SIMULATION   The representation of certain features of the behaviour or functioning of one system by means of actions of another, e.g. the representation of physical phenomena by the action of computers, or even a computer by another computer.
This term is also used in a different sense as an Operational Research technique in which the operation of a real system is represented by a simplified model.

SOFTWARE   Programs and procedures associated with a data processor in order to facilitate its use.

SOLID-STATE   An imprecise term used to denote components that depend on electric or magnetic phenomena in solids in contrast to those depending on phenomena in a vacuum or a rarefied gas, e.g. transistors and other semiconductor components and ferrite components.

SOURCE DOCUMENT   A document from which data is extracted, e.g. a document that contains typed or handwritten data to be key-punched.

STORE   Same as Memory.

STORE-AND-FORWARD   A special method of operating a network by which data is accumulated over a period of time at a message-switching

Glossary

centre for subsequent very high speed transmission.

SYSTEM — A set or arrangement of entities that forms, or is considered as, an organised whole.

Note: This term is a very general one that is applied to both hardware and software entities; therefore, it must be carefully qualified to be meaningful, e.g. computer system, management information system, number system.

TAPE CARTRIDGE — A container to hold magnetic tape. The tape forms an integral part of the cartridge that protects it and aids tape loading.

TAPE DECK — An equipment unit containing a tape transport mechanism together with reading and writing heads and associated electrical circuits used with magnetic tape.

TERMINAL — A point or device in a system or communications network at which data can either enter or leave.

TIME-SHARING —
1. The use of a given device by a number of other devices, one at a time, in rapid succession.
2. In automatic data processing the concept is that a certain functional unit, a part of the equipment, etc. is controlled in different periods of time and in rapid succession by various users, programs or other units, parts of equipment, etc. The sequence in which sharing takes place is controlled automatically and it can either be predetermined or can be arranged on a request basis, within a priority scheme or not.

TOUCH-TONE TELEPHONE — A telephone instrument so designed that it can be used for inputting small amounts of digital data accurately and rapidly into a computer system. Also known as keyphone.

TRANSLATOR	A program that translates from one language into another language. In the field of programming the term is commonly used in the more restricted sense of translation from one programming language to another.
UPDATING	The incorporation into a master file of the changes required to reflect recent transactions or other events.
VDU	*See* Visual Display (Unit).
VIDEOFILE	A document storage system allowing very large document collections to be held on special magnetic tape with the facility of rapid retrieval in the form of a visual display or hard copy.
VIEW-PHONE	A system that adds vision to normal telephone facilities. It may also be used as a visual display unit.
VISUAL DISPLAY UNIT (VDU)	An output device that presents data in a transient form (character or graphical) usually on the screen of a cathode-ray tube. It may form part of a remote data terminal system.
WORD	A group of bits or characters treated as a unit and capable of being stored in one storage cell.
(TO) WRITE	To record data in a store or data carrier.

Index

ACCUMULATOR, of automatic digital computer, 117–20, 123–7
Accuracy of data, 63, 64
Addition operation, 115
Address part, 120
ALGOL, 37, 39, 131
Algorithm, 22
Analogue computers, 32, 33
Analogue-to-digital conversion, 36, 44
Assembler, 130, 131
Autocode, 130, 131
Automatic Library Facility (ALF), 76 et seq
Automation—
 definition, 20
 difference from mechanisation, 15
 explanation, 15
 medical, 16, 23

BABBAGE, Charles, 125
Bacteria, identification of, 79 et seq
Batch made (processing), 12, 28
Binary, natural, 140–2
Binary language, 132–9
Biochemical laboratory, 101 et seq
Branching instruction, 126

CARD punch, 45
Card reader, 43
Central processor, 41, 48, 56, 115–20
Chess, using computer to play, 8, 12
'Clear' operation, 116
COBOL, 37, 39, 131
Codification, discussion, 67 et seq
Coding of data, necessity for, 65 et seq
Communications, Post Office lines, 53

Compiler, 130, 131, 146
Computer graphics, 47
Computer language, 130
Computer operations, elementary, 115–20
Computer system, general, 51, 52
Computers, physical attibutes, 136–9
CORAL, 37, 39

DATA preparation, 34
Decision-making process, 18, 19
Diagnosis, use of computers for, 9 et seq, 74, 85 et seq
Drugs, monitoring, 61

ECG, 105
EDSAC, 26
ENIAC, 24 et seq

FACTORY organisation, development of, 16
Ferrite core store, 26, 138
Figure-shift code, 137
Flow chart, 38, 39
FORTRAN, 37, 39, 131
Function part, 120

GRAPH plotter, 46, 108

HOSPITAL activity analysis, 62
Human brain, comparison with computer, 14

IDENTIFICATION of bacteria, 79 et seq
Immunisation schedule, 56, 57
Information loop, 21 22
Initial orders, 124
Input, 41
Input operation, 116
Instruction, 120
Interface, 22, 51
Interrogation of patients, 94 et seq

KEYBOARD punching, 137

LABORATORY automation, 11
Languages, high-level computer, 122, 129–32
Left shift operation, 116
Letter-shift code, 137
Line printer, 45, 53
Loop organisation, 128–9

MACHINE code, 122
Magnetic disc, 49
Magnetic drum, 50
Magnetic ink character reader, 43
Magnetic tape, 48, 56
  for surveys, 58, 59
Mark sensing, 44
Mechanisation, 17, 20
Medical records, 52, 55 et seq, 109
Mini-computers, 30
Monitoring drugs, 61
Morbidity survey, 63
Multi-phase screening, 100
Muscle power, comparison with computer power, 16 et seq

OBSTETRICS, 60
Optical character reader, 44
Order, 120
Order code, of computer, 124
Output, 41
Output operation, 116

PATIENT identification, 71 et seq
Patient monitoring, 11, 105
Patient records, 52, 55 et seq, 109
Pattern recognition, 106

Program—
  special, 124
  stored, 120–5
Program of instructions, 120
Programming, 120
  general explanation, 37
  in machine code, 122
Programming techniques, 125–9
Punched cards, 35, 43
Punched paper tape, 36, 43

RADIATION treatment planning, 5, 106 et seq
Register, 117

SIMULATION, modelling, 12, 111
Statistics—
  use of computer to analyse, 58, 59
  use of computer to determine significance of, 60
'Stop' instruction, 122
Sub-routines, library of, 129–30
Subtraction operation, 116
SWITCH, 68 et seq
System analysis, 40

TAPE punch, 45
Tape reader, 43
Teleprinter, 45, 53
Terminals—
  'intelligent', 54
  remote, explanation, 28
  remote, job entry 54
Time sharing systems, 27 et seq
Traffic control, 11 et seq
Transistors, 138
Translation by computer, 2, 7, 12
Treatment, 9 et seq
Two-state devices, 137

VISUAL display unit, 46, 108

'WORDS', 117
'Write' operation, 116

X-RAY reports, 66